CHINESE
MEDICINE
CURES

PMS

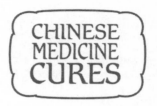

PMS

BOB FLAWS

Adapted for the UK by Sylvia Schroer

foulsham
LONDON • NEW YORK • TORONTO • SYDNEY

foulsham

The Publishing House, Bennetts Close,
Cippenham, Berkshire SL1 5AP, England

ISBN 0-572-02539-4

Printed in Great Britain by St. Edmundsbury Press, Bury St. Edmunds, Suffolk

CONTENTS

PREFACE

I have been practising traditional Chinese medicine for almost 20 years, and for 17 of those years I have been specialising in Chinese medical gynaecology. You could say that I have 'written the book' (actually ten or more) on all areas of Chinese gynaecology in English. No matter what other gynaecological diseases or complaints my patients may have, the vast majority also suffer from PMS (premenstrual syndrome). Based on my many years as a clinician, I can say without hesitation that traditional Chinese medicine treats PMS very well.

Although I have written numerous textbooks and clinical manuals for professionals on all aspects of Chinese gynaecology, up till now there has not been any simple discussion of the Chinese medical diagnosis and treatment of PMS written specifically for the layperson. Therefore, I have created this book for sufferers of PMS and their friends and families. Hopefully, the reader will find that traditional Chinese medicine is an enlightening and empowering alternative or complement to more conventional treatment. Chinese medicine has a holistic, centuries-old, well developed and coherent theory about the causes and treatment of PMS. Not only is this theory enlightening, providing as it does a perspective on this common complaint wholly different from that of modern Western medicine, it is also empowering. Based on this, women will find there are all sorts of things, most of which are free or very low cost, that they can do for themselves in order to relieve and even cure their PMS.

When I was a teenager, girls used to call their menstruation 'the curse', as if PMS and menstrual pain were simply the lot of all Eve's daughters. Chinese medicine says that this is not so. PMS does not need to occur, and if it does, Chinese medicine has ways to eliminate or minimise it.

Bob Flaws

INTRODUCTION

Denise was really fed up. She had been cranky and irritable for several days. She was snappish with her boyfriend and found herself in tears over the smallest of things. Partly, she was angry at herself for being so out of control. Her life was not all that bad. When her boyfriend had reluctantly asked her if her period was due in the next couple of days, she had really blown her top. They had had a big argument and he had walked out, slamming the door behind him. When he came back, he walked around the flat as if on eggshells. This only infuriated Denise all the more. Three days later, Denise's period did, in fact, begin. The next month, the same thing happened all over again.

Does this sound familiar? If so, this book may very well help you break the cycle of PMS. According to traditional Chinese medicine, PMS is most definitely classified as a valid gynaecological complaint or condition. The good news is that practitioners of Chinese medicine have been curing women's PMS for centuries, if not millennia.

This book is a layperson's guide to the diagnosis and treatment of PMS with Chinese medicine. In it, you will learn what causes PMS and what you can do about it. Hopefully, you will be able to recognise yourself and your symptoms in these pages. If you can see yourself in the signs and symptoms I discuss below, I feel confident I will be able to give you a number of self-help techniques that can minimise your monthly discomfort. As a specialist in the Chinese medical treatment of gynaecological complaints for 17 years, I know that Chinese medicine cannot cure every gynaecological disease, but when it comes to PMS, it is the best alternative I know. When a woman calls me and says that PMS is her major complaint, I know that, if she follows my advice, together we can cure or at least reduce her premenstrual signs and symptoms.

WHAT IS PMS?

PMS refers to a group of symptoms that occur at a specific time during the menstrual cycle. The symptoms typically include: nervousness, irritability, emotional instability, depression, headaches, oedema (fluid retention) and breast tenderness. It usually occurs seven to ten days before menstruation and disappears a few hours after the onset of menstrual flow although it may take several days to subside in some women. It is sometimes referred to as premenstrual tension or PMT. The symptoms of PMS can vary from woman to woman and, as we will see below, some women's PMS includes dozens of symptoms and complaints. According to Western medical literature, over 150 symptoms have been reported in association with PMS.

IS PMS REALLY A DISEASE?

Whilst some doctors may not be sympathetic to the fact that PMS is a disease as such, most doctors would agree that it can seriously disrupt a woman's life. Practitioners of Chinese medicine have realised for over 1,000 years that some women get certain symptoms cyclically before each menses. Recent studies have established that premenstrual changes, both psychological and physical, are organically based. This means that the signs and symptoms of PMS are related to chemical changes that occur in the body in the time before the onset of the monthly menstruation. As a clinician, I can assure women that PMS is very much a real complaint and that it is not 'all in the mind', although the mind most certainly does play an important role in both the cause and treatment of PMS.

Up to 80 per cent of women of reproductive age experience premenstrual emotional and physical changes. It is estimated that 20–40 per cent of these women experience some difficulty as a result of these changes during the days before the onset of a period, and 2.5–5 per cent of sufferers report a significant negative impact on their work, lifestyle or relationships.

There is currently no clinical or laboratory test to confirm a diagnosis of PMS. Rather, its diagnosis depends on the use of a menstrual calendar to track and verify the fact that a woman's signs and symptoms are definitely related to her menstrual cycle month after month.

WHAT CAUSES PMS?

There is no single clearly identified biological or physiological explanation for PMS. However, some Western doctors think PMS is to do with an oestrogen imbalance. Oestrogen is one of the two main hormones secreted by the ovaries that control the menstrual cycle, the other being progesterone. Oestrogen exerts a fluid-retaining action on body tissues, and fluid retention plays a part in some of the symptoms of PMS such as weight gain, oedema, abdominal bloating, breast tenderness and pain.

It has also been suggested that PMS is due to a vitamin B_6 deficiency, low blood sugar, and/or a high level of prolactin, the hormone that governs milk production. Another recent theory holds that PMS is caused by sudden changes in the levels of naturally occurring morphine-like substances in the brain. According to this theory, cyclical changes in female hormone levels produce fluctuations in the levels of these substances. First, a rise in these substances causes depression for a week to ten days before menstruation and then their sudden drop just before the onset of menstruation leads to nervousness and irritability. At the moment, there is no one theory that can explain all the signs and symptoms of PMS.

With regard to Western medicine, there are many unanswered questions about PMS. There really is no explanation as to why some women suffer from it so much more than others.

HOW WESTERN MEDICINE TREATS PMS

The first thing a doctor or GP would do would be to ascertain whether the PMS was tied in with difficult periods. If this was the case, and particularly in younger women, the first line of treatment is likely to be some kind of hormone manipulation such as the contraceptive pill. In older women who experienced a lot of symptoms to do with fluid retention, a diuretic such as bendrofluazide might be prescribed. If the emotional symptoms were very disruptive to a woman's life and were causing depression and anxiety, then the GP might treat this with antidepressants and possibly tranquillisers, although prescribing tranquillisers for this condition is not common due to their highly addictive nature. A good GP might also suggest trying vitamin supplements and/or evening primrose oil.

Western medicine cannot really offer a cure for PMS and all medication has side-effects. Chinese medicine is however able to alleviate PMS without side-effects; it offers a safe and effective alternative approach and, as we shall see, treats both the cause of PMS and the symptoms.

EAST IS EAST AND WEST IS WEST

In order for the reader to understand and make sense of the rest of this book on Chinese medicine and PMS, it is important to understand that the Chinese system of medical thought and practice is quite distinct and separate from modern Western medicine. This means shifting models of reality when it comes to thinking about Chinese medicine. It has taken the Chinese more than 2,000 years to develop this medical system. In fact, Chinese medicine is the oldest continually practised, literate, professional medicine in the world. It is best to approach Chinese medicine on its own terms rather than trying to explain it according to Western medical science.

Most people reading this book will have some basic knowledge of biology. Whether we recognise it or not, most of us Westerners think of what we learned about the human body at school as the one true description of reality, rather than as one possible description. If Chinese medicine is to make any sense to Westerners at all, we need to accept the notion that there may be other valid descriptions of the human body, its functions, health and disease. In grappling with this fundamentally important issue, it is useful to think about the concepts of a map and the terrain it describes.

If we take the United Kingdom as an example, we can have numerous different maps of this country's land mass. One map might show population. Another might show per capita incomes. Another might simply be a road map. We could also show political or county boundaries. In fact, there could be an infinite number of different maps of the United Kingdom depending on what one was trying to show and do. As long as the map is based on accurate information and has been created with self-consistent logic, then one map is not necessarily more correct than another. The issue is to use the right map for what you are trying to do. If you wanted to drive from London to Glasgow, then a road map is probably the best one for the job but it is not necessarily a truer or more real description of the United Kingdom than a map showing annual rainfall.

The point I am trying to make is that the map is not the terrain. The Western biological map of the human body is only one potentially useful medical map. It is no more true than the traditional Chinese medical map, and the facts of one map cannot be reduced to the criteria or standards of another unless they share the same logic right from the beginning. As long as the Western medical map is capable of solving a person's disease in a cost-effective, time-efficient manner without side-effects or iatrogenesis (illness caused by treatment), then it is a useful map. Chinese medicine needs to be judged in the same way. The Chinese medical map of health and disease is just as real and every bit as useful as the Western biological map as long as in using it practitioners and patients are able to solve health problems in a safe and effective way.

The following chapter is an introduction to the fundamental concepts of Chinese medicine. If you have a basic understanding of some of these fundamental concepts you will be able to appreciate how Chinese medicine may help in the treatment of PMS.

AN OVERVIEW OF THE CHINESE MEDICAL MAP

In this chapter, we will look at an overview of Chinese medicine. In particular, we will discuss yin and yang, qi, blood and essence, the viscera and bowels and the channels and network vessels. Then, in the following chapter, we will go on to see how Chinese medicine views the menstrual cycle and menstruation itself. After that, we will look at the Chinese medical diagnosis and treatment of a wide range of premenstrual signs and symptoms. Should you find any of the language or terms used to describe Chinese medicine difficult to understand, there is a glossary on page 157 to which you can refer.

YIN AND YANG

To understand Chinese medicine, one must first understand the concepts of yin and yang since these are the most basic concepts in this system. Yin and yang are the cornerstones for understanding, diagnosing and treating the body and mind in Chinese medicine. In a sense, all the other theories and concepts of Chinese medicine are simply an elaboration of yin and yang. Most people have probably already heard of yin and yang but might not have a clear idea of what these terms mean.

The concepts of yin and yang can be used to describe everything that exists in the universe, including all the parts and functions of the body. Originally, yin referred to the shady side of a hill and yang to the sunny side of the hill. Since sunshine and shade are two interdependent sides of a single reality, these two aspects of the hill are seen as part of a single whole. Other examples of yin and yang are that night exists only in relation to day, and cold exists only in relation to heat. According to Chinese thought, every single thing that exists in the universe has these two aspects, a yin and a yang. Thus everything has a front and a back, a top and a bottom, a left and a right, and a beginning and an end. However, something is yin or yang only in relation to its paired complement. Nothing is of itself yin or yang.

It is the concepts of yin and yang that make Chinese medicine a holistic medicine. This is because, based on this unitary and complementary vision of reality, no body part or body function is viewed as separate or isolated from the whole person. The table below shows a list of some yin and yang pairs as they apply to the body. As we can see from this list, it is possible to describe every aspect of the body in terms of yin and yang.

Yin	Yang
Form	Function
Organs	Bowels
Blood	Qi
Inside	Outside
Front of body	Back of body
Right side	Left side
Lower body	Upper body
Cool, cold	Warm, hot
Stillness	Activity, movement

QI AND BLOOD

Qi

Qi (pronounced chee) and blood are the most important complementary pairs of yin and yang within the human body. It is said that, in the world, yin and yang are water and fire, but in the human body, yin and yang are blood and qi. Qi is yang in relation to blood, which is yin. Qi is often translated as energy and certainly energy is a manifestation of qi. Chinese language scholars would say, however, that qi is larger than any single type of energy described by modern Western science. Paul Unschuld, perhaps one of the greatest living sinologists, translates the word qi as influences. This conveys the sense that qi is what is responsible for change and movement. Thus, within Chinese medicine, qi is that which motivates all movement and transformation or change.

In Chinese medicine, qi is defined as having five specific functions:

1. Defence

Qi is responsible for protecting the exterior of the body from invasion by external pathogens. This qi, called defensive qi, flows through the exterior or outer portion of the body.

2. Transformation

Qi transforms substances so that they can be utilised by the body. An example of this function is the transformation of the food we eat into nutrients to nourish the body, which then produces more qi and blood.

3. Warming

Qi, being relatively yang, is inherently warm, and one of the main functions of the qi is to warm the entire body, both inside and out. If this warming function of the qi is weak, then the lack of warmth and resulting cold may cause the flow of qi and blood to be congealed in a similar way to the cold's effect on water – freezing.

4. Restraint

Qi holds all the organs and substances of the body in their proper place. Thus all the organs, blood and fluids need qi to keep them from falling or leaking out of their specific pathways. If this function of the qi is weak, then problems like uterine prolapse, a tendency to bruise easily or urinary incontinence may occur.

5. Transportation

Qi provides the motivating force for all transportation and movement in the body. Every aspect of the body that moves is moved by the qi. Hence the qi moves the blood and body fluids throughout the body. It moves food through the stomach and blood through the vessels.

Blood

In Chinese medicine, just as in modern Western medicine, blood refers to the red fluid that flows through our vessels, but it also has different meanings and implications. Fundamentally, blood is the substance that nourishes and moistens all the body tissues. Without blood, body tissues cannot function properly. In addition, when there is insufficient blood or it is scanty, body tissues become dry and wither.

Qi and blood are closely interrelated. In Chinese medicine it is said, 'Qi is the commander of the blood and blood is the mother of qi.' This means that it is qi that moves the blood but that it is the blood that provides the nourishment and physical foundation for the creation and existence of the qi.

In Chinese medicine, blood provides the following functions for the body:

1. Nourishment

Blood nourishes the body. Along with qi, the blood goes to every part of the body. When the blood is deficient, function decreases and tissues atrophy or shrink.

2. Moistening

Blood moistens the body tissues. This includes the skin, eyes and ligaments and tendons, or what are simply called the sinews of the body in Chinese medicine. Blood deficiency can cause drying out and consequent stiffening of various body tissues throughout the body.

3. Material foundation for the spirit or mind

In Chinese medicine, the mind and body are considered as one. The blood (yin) supplies the material support and nourishment for the mind (yang), allowing it to become 'bright' (i.e. conscious and clever), and stay rooted in the body. If the blood is insufficient, the mind can 'float', causing problems like insomnia, agitation and unrest.

ESSENCE

Along with qi and blood, essence is one of the three most important constituents of the body. Essence is the most fundamental, essential material the body uses for its growth, maturation and reproduction. There are two forms of this essence. We inherit essence from our parents and we also produce our own essence from the food and drink that we consume and the air we breathe.

The essence that comes from our parents is what determines our basic constitution, strength and vitality. We each have a finite, limited amount of this inherited essence. It is important to protect and conserve this essence because all bodily functions depend upon it and when it is gone we die.

The depletion of essence has serious implications for our overall health and well-being. Fortunately, the essence derived from food and drink helps to bolster and support this inherited essence. So, if we eat well and do not consume more qi and blood than we create each day, then when we sleep at night, this surplus qi, and more especially blood, is transformed into essence.

THE VISCERA AND BOWELS

In Chinese medicine, the internal organs (called viscera so as not to become confused with the Western biological entities of the same name) have a much wider area of function and influence than in Western medicine. Each viscus has distinct responsibilities for maintaining the physical and psychological health of the individual. From a Chinese medical perspective it is more useful to view each viscus as a sphere of influence or a network that spreads throughout the body, rather than as the distinct and separate physical organ that is described by Western science. It is for this reason that the renowned German sinologist, Manfred Porkert, refers to the viscera as orbs rather than as organs. In Chinese medicine, the relationship between the various viscera and other parts of the body is facilitated by the channel and network vessel system that we will discuss later.

According to Chinese medicine, there are five main viscera that are relatively yin and six main bowels that are relatively yang. The five yin viscera are the heart, lungs, liver, spleen and kidneys. The six yang bowels are the stomach, small intestine, large intestine, gall bladder, urinary bladder and a system that Chinese medicine refers to as the triple burner. All the functions of the entire body are subsumed or described under these eleven organs or spheres of influence. Thus Chinese medicine as a system does not have a pancreas, a pituitary gland or ovaries, as their functions and others are described by the sphere of influence of the five viscera and six bowels. The actual functions of the viscera and bowels are more important and wider-reaching than their physical structure. For example, someone who has had their gall bladder removed will still have available to them many of the functional aspects of the gall bladder as regarded by Chinese medicine. This would obviously not be the case with organs essential to survival, such as the heart and lungs, but their functional aspects are still much wider-reaching according to Chinese medicine.

Within this system, the five viscera are the most important. These are the organs that Chinese medicine says are responsible for the creation and transformation of qi and blood and the storage of essence. For instance, the kidneys are responsible for the excretion of urine, but in addition they have many other areas of responsibility or spheres of influence such as hearing, the strength of the bones, sex, reproduction, maturation and growth, the lower and upper back and the lower legs in general and the knees in particular.

The Chinese viscera may have the same name and even some overlapping functions but they are quite different from the organs of modern Western medicine. Each of the five Chinese medical viscera also has a corresponding tissue, sense, spirit and emotion related to it. These are outlined in the table below.

Organ	Tissue	Sense	Spirit	Emotion
Lungs	Skin/body hair	Smell	Corporeal soul	Grief/sadness
Spleen	Flesh	Taste	Thought	Thinking/worry
Kidneys	Bones/head hair	Hearing	Will	Fear
Liver	Sinews	Sight	Ethereal soul	Anger
Heart	Blood vessels	Speech	Spirit	Joy/fright

In addition, each Chinese medical viscus or bowel possesses both a yin and a yang aspect. The yin aspect of a viscus or bowel refers to its substantial nature or tangible form. Further, an organ's yin is responsible for the nurturing, cooling and moistening of that viscus or bowel. The yang aspect of the viscus or bowel represents its functional activities or what it does. An organ's yang aspect is also warming. When balanced, these two aspects, yin and yang, form and function, cooling and heating, create good health. If either yin or yang becomes too strong or too weak, the resulting imbalance may lead to disease.

The kidneys

In Chinese medicine, the kidneys are considered to be the foundation of our life. Since the developing foetus is shaped like a kidney and because the kidneys are the main viscus for the storage of inherited essence, the kidneys are referred to as the prenatal root. Keeping the kidney qi strong and kidney yin and yang in relative balance is considered essential to good health and longevity. According to Chinese medicine, the kidneys are actively involved in:

1. Human reproduction, development and maturation

These are the same functions we used when describing the essence. This is because the essence is stored in the kidneys. Health problems related to reproduction, development and maturation are considered to be problems of the kidney essence. Excessive sexual activity, drug use, or prolonged over-exhaustion can all damage and consume kidney essence. Kidney essence is also consumed by the simple act of ageing.

2.Water metabolism

The kidneys work in co-ordination with the lungs and spleen to ensure that water is spread properly throughout the body and that excess water is excreted as urine. Problems such as oedema (swelling caused by water retention), excessive dryness or excessive day- or night-time urination can indicate a weakness of kidney function.

3. Hearing
As was previously mentioned, each of the viscera is associated with a particular sense organ. The kidneys are associated with the ears and auditory problems such as diminished hearing and ringing in the ears can therefore be due to kidney weakness.

4. The grasping of qi
This means that one of the functions of the kidney qi is to 'pull down' or absorb the breath from the lungs and 'root' it in the lower abdomen. Certain types of asthma and chronic cough are the result of a weakness in this kidney function.

5. Bones and marrow
The kidneys are associated with bones and marrow, which means that problems of the bones, such as osteoporosis, degenerative disc disease and weak legs and knees, can all reflect a kidney imbalance.

6. Yin and yang
Kidney yin and yang are the foundation for the yin and yang of all the other organs and bowels and body tissues of the entire body. This concept illustrates the importance of the kidneys as the root or foundation of our life and all the body's energies. If either kidney yin or yang is deficient, eventually the yin or yang of the other viscera and bowels will become deficient.

7. Storing the will

Will in this sense refers to will-power and desire. If kidney qi is deficient, these aspects of our human nature can be weakened. Conversely, pushing ourselves to extremes both physically and mentally can eventually exhaust our kidneys.

8. Fear

There is a relationship between the kidneys and fear. Fear can manifest when the kidney qi is deficient. Conversely, excessive fear can damage and weaken the kidneys.

9. The lower back

There is a relationship between the health of the kidneys and the lower back, which Chinese medicine refers to as the mansion of the kidneys. If the kidneys are weak, then there may be lower back pain or soreness.

The liver

The liver is associated with the flow of blood and qi throughout the body. According to Chinese medicine, emotions are also related to the flow of qi so the liver is considered to be very important to the expression and flow of the emotions. The liver is also important to the process of digestion and because of its relationship with the flow of blood it is very much tied up with menstruation. As we will see in the following chapters, the liver is fundamental to the Chinese medical diagnosis and treatment of PMS. The basic Chinese medical aspects that relate to the liver include:

1. Coursing and discharge

These terms refer to the uninhibited spreading of qi to every part of the body. If the liver is not able to maintain the free and smooth flow of qi throughout the body, multiple physical and emotional symptoms can develop. This function of the liver is most easily damaged by emotional causes, especially by anger and frustration. If the liver is stressed due to pent-up anger, the flow of qi can become depressed or stagnate.

This is called liver qi stagnation and it can lead to a wide range of health problems, including PMS, chronic digestive disturbance and depression. It is essential to keep our liver qi flowing freely throughout the body.

2. Storing the blood

The liver regulates the amount of blood in circulation. In particular, when the body is at rest, such as during sleep, the blood in the extremities returns to the liver. Due to the relationship with the blood, the liver is said to be yin in form but yang in function. This means the liver requires enough blood to keep it and its associated tissues (the sinews) moist and supple, cool and relaxed.

3. Controlling the sinews

The sinews refer mainly to the tendons and ligaments in the body. As mentioned above, the proper functioning of the tendons and ligaments depends upon the nourishment of liver blood to keep them moist and supple.

4. The eyes

The eyes are the specific sense organ corresponding to the liver. Therefore, according to Chinese medicine, many eye problems are related to the liver.

5. Anger

Inappropriate anger is the emotion that typically arises when the liver is diseased and when its qi does not flow freely. Anger, like all our emotions, is essential to our health and well-being. Learning how to listen to anger within ourselves and in turn use its powerful energy to transform our lives is a life-long challenge. Having a healthy liver is really important in regard to this. If anger is not dealt with, it can turn into rage, frustration and depression. If there is stagnation of qi in the liver, then it will be all the more likely that we experience these negative forms of anger. Anger and frustration can also damage the liver.

The heart

According to Chinese medicine, the heart is the emperor of the body and mind. When it comes to disease and illness, however, it generally plays a secondary rather than primary role. Rather than the heart initiating the disease, the disease, if it endures for a long time, will eventually affect the heart. This is particularly true in terms of PMS. Generally another viscus or bowel is affected before the heart. The specific aspects relating to the heart in Chinese medicine are:

1. Governing the blood

This means that it is the heart qi that 'stirs' or moves the blood within its vessels. This is roughly analogous to the idea of the heart pumping the blood in Western medicine. The pulsation of the blood through the arteries due to the contraction of the heart is referred to as the 'stirring of the pulse'. In fact, the Chinese word for pulse and vessel is the same. So this could also be translated as the 'stirring of the vessels'.

2. Storing the spirit

The spirit in this context refers to the mind. Therefore, this statement underscores that mental function, mental clarity and mental equilibrium are all associated with the heart. If the heart does not receive enough qi or blood or if the heart is disturbed by something, the spirit may become restless and this may produce symptoms of mental–emotional unrest, heart palpitations, insomnia, profuse dreams, etc.

3. Governing the vessels
This concept is very close to point 1 on page 26. The vessels refer to the blood vessels and also to the pulse.

4. Governing speech
If heart function becomes abnormal, this may be reflected in various speech problems, including raving and delirious speech, muttering to oneself and speaking incoherently.

5. The tongue
Since the heart has a special relationship with the tip of the tongue, heart problems may manifest as sores on the tip of the tongue.

6. Joy
The particular emotion associated with the heart is that of joy. Joy is a very healing emotion and can make the blood and qi flow more smoothly in the body; it can also harmonise other emotions if they become chaotic or overwhelming. However, should someone experience 'too much joy', i.e. too much excitement, this can be detrimental to the heart and can cause problems with the Chinese medical functions of the heart in terms of governing the blood and storing the spirit. Shock will also damage the heart.

The spleen
In Chinese medicine, the spleen plays a pivotal role in the creation of qi and blood and in the circulation and transformation of body fluids. Its role is very wide-reaching and more important than in Western medicine. This is an excellent illustration of how these two systems of medicine differ in their views of the internal organs and their functions. According to Chinese medicine the main functions of the spleen that relate to PMS are:

1. Movement and transformation
This refers to the movement and transformation of foods and liquids, i.e. the process of digestion. It may also refer to the movement and transformation of body fluids through the body. The spleen qi is largely responsible for controlling liquid metabolism in the body.

2. Restraining the blood
As mentioned above, one of the five functions of the qi is to restrain the fluids of the body, including the blood, within their proper channels and reservoirs. If the spleen qi is healthy and abundant, then the blood is held within its vessels properly. However, if the spleen qi becomes weak and insufficient, then the blood may flow outside its channels and vessels, resulting in various types of pathological bleeding, including those associated with the menstrual cycle.

3. Storing the constructive
The constructive is one of the types of qi in the body. Specifically, it is the qi responsible for nourishing and constructing the body and its tissues. This constructive qi is closely associated with the process of digestion and the creation of qi and blood from food and liquids. If the spleen fails to store, or runs out of, constructive qi, then the person becomes hungry and eventually fatigued.

4. Governing the muscles and flesh
This function is closely allied to the previous one. The constructive qi constructs or nourishes the muscles and flesh. If there is sufficient spleen qi producing sufficient constructive qi, then the person's body is well fleshed and rounded. In addition, their muscles are normally strong. Conversely, if the spleen becomes weak, this may lead to emaciation and/or lack of strength.

5. Governing the limbs

This means that the strength and function of the arms and legs is closely associated with the spleen. If the spleen is healthy and strong, then there is sufficient strength in their limbs and warmth in the four extremities. If the spleen becomes weak and insufficient, then there may be lack of strength in the limbs and lack of warmth or even tingling and numbness in their extremities.

6. The mouth

Just as the ears are the portals of the kidneys, the eyes are the portal of the liver and the tongue is the portal of the heart, the mouth is the portal of the spleen. Therefore, spleen disease often manifests as problems of the mouth, such as sores or bleeding from the gums.

7. Thought

In the West, we do not usually think of the process of thought as an emotion but in Chinese medicine thought is the emotion associated with the spleen. Perhaps it is better understood as worry or overthinking. This causes the spleen qi to bind, meaning that the spleen qi does not flow harmoniously; this typically manifests as loss of appetite, abdominal bloating after meals, and indigestion.

8. Engenderment and transformation

These terms refer to the creation or production of the qi and blood from the food and drink we take in each day. If the spleen receives and then properly transforms adequate food and drink, it engenders or creates qi and blood. The kidneys and lungs also participate in the creation of the qi, while the kidneys and heart also participate in the creation of the blood, but the spleen is the pivotal viscus in both processes, and spleen qi weakness and insufficiency is one of the main causes of qi and blood insufficiency and weakness.

The lungs

The lungs are not one of the main Chinese viscera involved in the causes of PMS. However, like the heart, the lungs often bear the brunt of disease processes initiated in other viscera and bowels. Called 'the delicate viscus', they are the most vulnerable of all the viscera and bowels, and are the most easily invaded by external pathogens. This is the Chinese explanation for the prevalence of colds and flu in comparison with other types of diseases.

As in Western medicine, the lungs are often subject to externally invading pathogens resulting in respiratory tract diseases. According to Chinese medicine, they are like a tent, known as 'the florid canopy', spreading over the top of all the other viscera and bowels. They are the first viscus to be assaulted by external pathogens invading the body from the top. Pathogenic qi moving upwards in the body eventually may accumulate in and affect the lungs. The lungs' sphere of influence also includes the skin and fluid metabolism. The main aspects of the functions of the lungs in Chinese medicine are:

1. Governing the qi

The lungs govern the downward spread and circulation of the qi. The lung qi moves all the rest of the qi in the body out to the edges and from the top of the body downwards. You could describe it as a sprinkler spraying out qi. This downward qi ensures body fluids are moved throughout the body, down to the kidneys and bladder and, eventually, out of the body.

2. The skin and hair

The skin and body hair correspond with the lungs. If the lungs become diseased, this often manifests as skin problems.

3. The voice

If there is sufficient lung qi, the voice is strong and clear. If there is insufficient lung qi, then the voice is weak and the person tries not to speak as a way of conserving their energy.

4. Regulating the water passageways

This statement emphasises the lung qi's role in moving body fluids outwards and downwards throughout the body, to arrive ultimately at the urinary bladder. If the lung qi fails to maintain the free flow and regulation of the water passageways, then fluids will collect and transform into dampness, producing oedema (swelling due to water retention).

5. The defensive exterior

I said above that the qi defends the body against invasion by external pathogens. In Chinese medicine, the exterior or outermost layer of the body is the area where the defensive qi circulates and the location where this defence takes place. The lungs govern this defensive qi. If the lungs function normally and there is sufficient defensive qi, then the body cannot be invaded by external pathogens. If the lungs are weak and the defensive qi is insufficient, then external pathogens may easily invade the exterior of the body, causing complaints such as colds, flu and allergies.

8. Mucus

Nasal mucus has to do, at least in part, with lung function. If the lungs are functioning correctly, there should not be any runny nose or nasal congestion.

9. The nose
Diseases or problems associated with the nose and its function are often associated with the Chinese medical concept of the lungs.

The bowels
According to Chinese medicine, the viscera are relatively more important than the bowels. Each viscus is paired with a bowel in a yin–yang relationship. The kidneys are paired with the urinary bladder, the liver is paired with the gall bladder, the heart is paired with the small intestine, the spleen is paired with the stomach, and the lungs are paired with the large intestine. In the case of the urinary bladder, gall bladder and stomach, these bowels receive their qi from their paired viscus and function very much as an extension of that viscus. The relationship between the other two viscera and bowels is not as close.

Above I mentioned that there are five viscera and six bowels. The sixth bowel is called the triple burner. It is said in Chinese: 'The triple burner has a function but no form'. The name triple burner refers to the three main areas of the torso. The upper burner is the chest. The middle burner is the space from the bottom of the rib cage to the level of the navel. The lower burner is the lower abdomen below the navel. These three spaces are called burners because all of the functions and transformations of the viscera and bowels that they contain are 'warm' transformations similar to the process of food cooking in a pot on a stove or chemical transformation in a furnace. On a physical level, the triple burner is really a generalised concept of how the other viscera and bowels function together as an organic unit in terms of the digestion of foods and liquids and the circulation and transformation of body fluids.

The channels and network vessels

Each viscus and bowel has a corresponding channel or meridian with which it is connected. In Chinese medicine, the inside of the body is made up of the viscera and bowels. The outside of the body is composed of the sinews, bones, muscles, flesh, skin and hair. The channels and network vessels (i.e. smaller connecting vessels) connect the inside to the outside of the body and it is through these channels and network vessels that the viscera and bowels connect with their corresponding body tissues.

The channel and network vessel system is a unique feature of traditional Chinese medicine. These channels and vessels are different from the circulatory, nervous or lymphatic systems. The earliest reference to these channels and vessels is in *Nei Jing (The Inner Classic)*, a text written around the second or third century BC.

The channels and vessels perform two basic functions. They are the pathways by which the qi and blood circulate through the body and between the organs and tissues. Additionally, as mentioned above, the channels connect the viscera and bowels internally with the exterior part of the body. This channel and vessel system functions in the body much like an information or communication network. The channels allow the various parts of our body to co-operate and interact to maintain our lives.

This channel and network vessel system is quite complex. There are 12 primary channels, six yin and six yang, each with a specific pathway through the external body and connected with an internal organ (see diagram overleaf). There are also extraordinary vessels, sinew channels, channel divergences, main network vessels and ultimately countless finer and finer network vessels permeating the entire body. All of these form a closed loop or circuit similar to, but distinct from, the Western circulatory system.

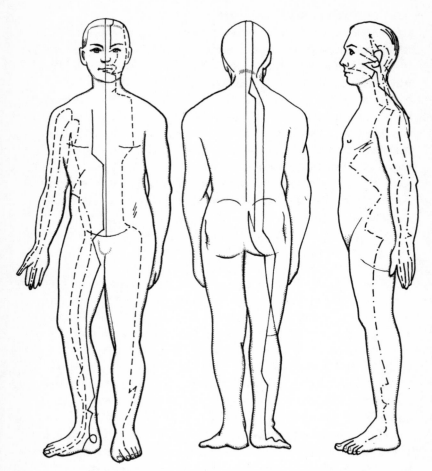

Acupuncture points are places located on the major channels where there is a special concentration of qi and blood. Because of the relatively greater quantity of qi and blood accumulated at these places, the sites act as switches that can control the flow of qi and blood in the channel on which the point is located. By stimulating these points in any of a number of different ways, one can speed up or slow down, make more or reduce, warm or cool down the qi and blood flowing in the channels and vessels. The main ways of stimulating these points and thus adjusting the flow of qi and blood in the channels and vessels are to manipulate them with acupuncture (see page 82) and to heat them by moxibustion (see page 126). Other commonly used ways of stimulating these points, and thus adjusting the qi and blood flowing through the channels and vessels, are massage, cupping, the application of magnets and the application of various herbal medicinals. If the channels and vessels are the pathways over which the qi and blood flow, then the acupuncture points are the places where this flow can be adjusted.

THE MENSTRUAL CYCLE IN CHINESE MEDICINE

It is said in Chinese medicine that men and women are basically the same. However, women have a uterus and thus they menstruate and can conceive, give birth and lactate. The menses themselves are a discharge of blood. For this discharge to take place, two things have to occur. First, a superabundance of blood must accumulate in the uterus for it eventually to spill over as the menstruate. Secondly, the qi and blood must be freely and uninhibitedly flowing in order to allow this brimming over. This means that, in order to understand menstruation, one must understand how blood is created and what might affect the free and uninhibited flow of qi and blood.

THE CREATION OF BLOOD

There are three viscera that participate in the creation of the blood. These are the kidneys, spleen and heart. The heart is the place where the blood is 'turned red' or finally created. However, first the spleen must send up the finest essence of food and liquids extracted in the process of digestion. If the spleen does not do this there will be insufficient supplies for the heart to transform these into blood. In addition, the kidneys must send up some essence to participate in the creation of blood.

So, if the kidneys lack sufficient essence, if the spleen fails to digest the finest essence of food and liquids and send this upwards, or if the heart, for any reason, cannot fulfil its function of 'turning the blood red', then there may be insufficient creation of blood. In addition, it is the heart's job to spread the blood to the rest of the body and eventually move it down to the uterus. It is said in Chinese medicine that the blood first goes to nourish and moisten the viscera and bowels and then it goes into the channels and vessels. From there it nourishes and moistens the rest of the tissues of the body and what collects in the uterus is what is left over after the blood has performed all these other jobs. When enough blood collects in the uterus to fill it, it overflows as the menses. Typically, a young to middle-aged, healthy woman will produce such a superabundance accumulating in the uterus once every 28–30 days.

THE CONTROL OF THE BLOOD

Although normal menstruation cannot occur if there is insufficient blood accumulated in the uterus, it can occur either too early or too late if the flow of blood is not controlled properly. Just as there are three viscera that engender and transform the blood, there are three viscera that govern or control the blood. These are the heart, liver and spleen. It is said that the heart qi governs the blood. Earlier we saw that this means that it is the heart qi that 'stirs' or pushes the blood. If the heart qi does not move the blood, the blood cannot move on its own. Thus it is said: 'If the qi moves, the blood moves. If the qi stops, the blood stops.'

In actual fact, the heart gets its qi primarily from the spleen. So a sufficiency of spleen qi is necessary for there to be enough heart qi to move the blood. In addition, the spleen qi restrains and contains the blood within its channels and vessels. If the spleen qi is too weak, it may allow the blood to seep out prematurely, or it may not cut off menstruation when it should. Finally, the liver stores the blood. It is the liver's job to regulate the amount of blood in circulation and it is liver qi that performs this function. If the liver qi spreads freely, then the blood moves. If the liver qi becomes depressed and stagnant, then the blood will also eventually become depressed and static.

It can be difficult at first to distinguish the difference between the spleen and the liver's role in maintaining the free and uninhibited flow of blood. The spleen qi ultimately (via the heart) provides the motivating force behind the propulsion of the blood but the liver allows the blood to flow freely through its channels and vessels. Think of it like this: if you have petrol in your car and the car is in good working order, you have the power to move the car. However, if you are stopped at a red light, you may not have the permission to move the car even though the power is there. In terms of the heart, spleen and liver, the flow of blood is the same. The heart and spleen provide the motivating power, but it is the liver qi that governs whether that blood flows freely or not.

If, for any reason, one of these three viscera does not function correctly in terms of the flow of blood, this may impede the free and timely flow of the menstruate.

THE FOUR PHASES OF THE MENSTRUAL CYCLE

Chinese medicine divides the menstrual cycle into four periods, each of roughly seven days. Phase one begins on the day the menses end. If one counts the days of the menstrual cycle from the first day of the onset of menstruation, this means that phase one typically begins on day four, five, six or seven. The uterus has discharged its accumulated blood and this leaves the body relatively empty or 'vacuous' of blood. Since blood is created at least in part out of kidney essence, and since, compared to yang qi, essence is a type of yin substance, during phase one, the body busies itself with making more yin and blood to replenish what was discharged.

Therefore, in Chinese gynaecology, we say that phase one corresponds to yin and the emphasis in the body is on replenishing yin blood.

Phase two corresponds to the days surrounding ovulation. Up till now, the body has been replenishing its yin. However, for ovulation to occur, yin must transform into yang. This transformation of yin into yang corresponds to the rise in basal body temperature that occurs after ovulation. If there is insufficient yin, it cannot transform into yang. Conversely, if there is insufficient yang, it cannot transform yin. In addition, if either the qi or the blood is not flowing freely, this transformation may also be impeded. Generally, phase two corresponds to days 10–16 in the monthly cycle and it corresponds to yang in the same way that phase one corresponds to yin.

Phase three corresponds to the premenstruum and to the qi. For things to go as they should in the woman's body, yang qi must stay strong for long enough and the qi must flow freely and in the right directions. Many of the signs and symptoms of PMS have to do with the yang qi not being strong enough or the qi (and therefore the blood) not flowing freely. Phase three may be counted from day 17 to the day before menstruation, i.e. day 28, and corresponds to qi.

Phase four is the menstruation itself. Since the onset of menstruation is counted as day one in the cycle, phase four may last anything from one or two days to six or seven, depending on the individual woman's constitution and age. Since, according to Chinese medicine, menstruation is a downward discharge of blood, phase four corresponds to the blood.

When looked at from this perspective, the menstrual cycle is made up of four (not always equal) segments corresponding to yin, yang, qi and blood. This relationship is shown in the chart overleaf.

Qi, blood, yin and yang
in relation to the menstrual cycle

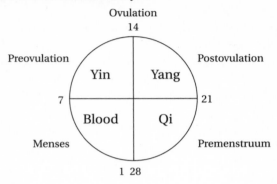

Problems may occur in any of these four phases and may occur for reasons other than the dominant correspondence in that phase. However, when a problem occurs in any of these four phases, the practitioner of Chinese medicine will first investigate to see if the dominant correspondence, i.e. yin, yang, qi or blood, is behaving as it should at that time. Since PMS occurs in the premenstruum, or phase three, most premenstrual complaints are attributed, either directly or indirectly, to problems with the flow of qi.

AGE AND THE MENSTRUAL CYCLE

In Chinese medicine, everything about the patient is taken into account. This includes their bodily constitution, their temperament, their lifestyle and occupation and their age. There is a famous saying in Chinese gynaecology: 'In adolescent (girls), blame the kidneys. In middle-aged (women), blame the liver. In older (women), blame the spleen.'

When adolescent girls first begin menstruating, their cycles are often irregular. They may go several months or more between menses and their periods may not come regularly every 28–30 days until several years after the beginning of menstruation. In Chinese medicine, this is explained as being due to the immaturity of the kidneys. Since the kidneys must supply essence to create the superabundance of blood necessary for menstruation to occur naturally, if the kidneys are not mature, they may not supply the needed essence every 28 days. Maturation is a process, not an all-or-nothing affair, so the amount of essence and, therefore, the regularity of the menstrual cycle, may fluctuate for some time before it becomes stable.

Once the kidneys have become stable and mature and menstruation occurs on a regular basis, then most gynaecological problems are due to an imbalance in the liver. In Chinese medicine, the liver is called the 'temperamental viscus'. This means that it is easily damaged or upset by emotional influences. In particular, it is said, 'The liver likes orderly reaching.' This means that the liver qi likes to spread out without restriction or hindrance, like a large broad-leafed tree. When the liver encounters frustration, its coursing and discharging of the qi is inhibited. The qi cannot flow as freely as it wants and it becomes depressed and stagnant. The qi becomes bottled up and this gives rise to inappropriate anger and irritability – anger is the emotion associated with Chinese liver problems.

When the qi becomes depressed and blocked, it affects the flow of blood and body fluids, because it is the qi that moves and transforms both of these. Menstruation is the discharge of blood and this discharge requires the free flow of qi in order to occur normally. Consequently, if the qi becomes depressed, the blood does not move, and if the blood does not move, menstruation cannot occur normally.

Dealing with life's ups and downs affects our emotions and therefore our liver's ability to spread the qi freely. It is unlikely that anyone in the modern world will go through life without a certain amount of liver qi stagnation and in women, this almost always causes some menstrual irregularity.

According to *Nei Jing (The Inner Classic)*, the spleen and stomach begin to decline at around 35 years of age. Since the spleen and its helper, the stomach, form the source of the creation of qi and blood from the food and liquids we consume, this decline in spleen–stomach function corresponds to a decline in the amounts of qi and blood produced.

This means that, from approximately 35 years of age till menopause, the spleen must struggle to produce enough qi and blood to nourish and empower the entire body and create a surplus of blood to flow over as the menstruate. This puts a heavy burden on the spleen and causes many women to show pronounced or more pronounced signs and symptoms of spleen weakness after the mid-30s and through the 40s. In such cases, the liver depression qi stagnation does not automatically go away. In fact, as we will see below, it may even get worse. However, this liver depression qi stagnation may not produce as many signs and symptoms as the spleen vacuity or weakness.

As we will see in the next chapter, PMS does not occur without liver depression qi stagnation. However, as a woman moves into her mid-30s and through her 40s, PMS is not just due to the liver but also due to the spleen and the other viscera and bowels associated with the spleen and liver, most notably the heart and kidneys. Therefore, we need to consider the influence of age in attempting to understand the causes and treatment of PMS from a Chinese medical perspective, and why it often gets worse, not better, in women as they age.

MENOPAUSE AND CHINESE MEDICINE

Eventually, the body in its wisdom recognises it is not healthy to try to create qi and blood to nourish and empower the rest of the body at the same time as continuing to menstruate regularly with the loss of blood that that necessarily entails. Therefore, the body initiates a transformation which, from the Chinese medical point of view, is literally a 'change in life'. The Chinese medical literature does not say exactly how, but at some point, the heart ceases sending blood down to collect in the uterus. Just as maturation does not happen all at once, this process is also a gradual one in most women. Periods do not just suddenly stop. Menopause is commonly preceded by months or even years of a certain amount of menstrual irregularity. Eventually, the heart stops sending blood down to the uterus. This means the kidneys are now free to send essence up to accumulate in the heart, where it joins with the qi and blood sent up by the spleen and becomes 'spirit'.

A woman therefore makes a transition from being a mother of babies to becoming a mother of her tribe, the *femme sage* or wise woman full of spirit. If this change occurs smoothly, it naturally puts an end to any PMS, since the woman no longer has any periods. The smooth cessation of menstruation is, like all other transformations in the body, dependent on the free flow of liver qi. Since PMS and liver depression qi stagnation are so closely linked, there is a strong correlation between menopausal complaints, PMS and liver depression qi stagnation. The more a woman suffers from PMS, the more likely she is to have problems in the menopause. In other words, PMS and menopausal syndrome are ultimately not two separate diseases but a continuum whose core issue is liver depression qi stagnation. We will discuss this transition from PMS into menopausal complaints in greater detail below, but more information about Chinese medicine and menopause is contained in *Menopause, A Second Spring: Making a Smooth Transition with Chinese Medicine* (see page 150).

THE CHINESE MECHANISMS OF PMS

Although Chinese medicine has recognised and developed treatments for premenstrual complaints for centuries, if not millennia, PMS as a modern disease concept is a relatively recent addition to the Chinese medical literature. In the Chinese language, premenstrual syndrome is frequently translated as *jing xing xian qi zhu zheng*. *Jing xing* means menstrual movement; *xian qi* means before the period, and *zhu zheng* means various pathological conditions, or syndrome. This is an attempt to translate PMS literally into Chinese. This new category is now beginning to show up in Chinese gynaecology texts and articles. However, listed in the table of contents of the gynaecology section of the *Yi Zong Jin Jian (The Golden Mirror of Ancestral Medicine)*, the famous Qing dynasty compendium of medicine published in 1749 AD, under the subheading of 'regulating menstruation', there are a group of conditions each prefixed by the words *jing xing*. These words mean menstrual movement. The implication is that in Chinese these conditions are all in some way concerned with pathological mechanisms occurring when the menstrual blood is moving to and out of the uterus. So in the older Chinese medical literature, these *jing xing* diseases refer to what we now group as the various conditions constituting premenstrual syndrome.

The list of such menstrual movement conditions is extensive. Although some Chinese gynaecology texts give only one or two menstrual movement diseases, others give dozens. We could really say that any complaint or pathological condition occurring during the premenstruum or the menses themselves (including the 150 PMS symptoms recognised by Western medicine) can be prefixed with the words 'menstrual movement'. This means that there are some more commonly seen menstrual movement diseases and there are some pretty unusual ones. When I teach Chinese medicine practitioners how to diagnose and treat PMS, I ask the women in the audience to name all the various complaints they know, either from their own or their patients' experience to occur premenstrually. Listed below is a typical sample:

Irritability
Tendency to cry easily
Impaired memory
Lack of concentration
Lack of clear thinking
Fatigue
Loss of co-ordination
Swollen, tender breasts
Growth of cystic lumps in the breasts
Oedema of the face, hands and feet
Lower abdominal distension
Lower abdominal cramping
Lack of strength
Headaches, including migraines
Catching a cold or flu
Cravings for sweets
Cravings for salt
Cravings for carbohydrates
Increased appetite in general
Lack of appetite
Insomnia
Night sweats
Lower back pain
Acne
Hives
Vaginitis and vaginal sores
Heart palpitations
Diarrhoea

Nausea and vomiting
Constipation
Flatulence
Painful and/or frequent urination
Loss of libido
Spotting of blood
Nosebleeds
Coughing or vomiting blood
Blood in the urine or stools
Worsening of eczema or psoriasis
Cold sores

Any of these complaints can and do occur cyclically during the premenstruum in some women. When they occur on a regular basis before each menstruation, they are prefaced by the words 'menstrual movement', as in 'menstrual movement diarrhoea' or 'menstrual movement hives'. Most women with PMS will have several of these complaints. It is the fact that PMS does include more than a single complaint or symptom that it is called a syndrome, remembering that in Chinese, syndrome is translated as 'various conditions'.

So any abnormal discomfort or complaint can be labelled as PMS according to Chinese medicine. More unusual complaints discussed in the Chinese medical literature include menstrual movement pneumothorax (a lung condition causing chest pain and shortness of breath) and menstrual movement lip swelling and pain. The sole criteria for a complaint to be labelled as a menstrual movement disease in Chinese medicine is that it must occur on a regular basis before or during the menses.

This means that PMS in modern Chinese gynaecology does not focus on one particular issue. The actual symptoms that any given patient may present are highly variable and idiosyncratic.

To begin with, however, we shall examine the common textbook patterns associated with PMS in the contemporary Chinese gynaecology textbook literature. Both Sun Jiu-ling, author of *Fu Ke Zheng Zhi (Gynaecological Patterns and Treatments)* (see page 163) and Zhu Cheng-han, author of *Zhong Yi Fu Ke (Chinese Medical Gynaecology)* (see page 166), list PMS as a disease category similar to that in modern Western medicine. Sun discusses three patterns in the traditional Chinese medicine treatment of PMS. To these same three, Zhu adds a fourth. Understanding these four basic patterns will enable the practitioner and patient to understand the mechanisms behind most of the various signs and symptoms associated with PMS. I will give several more in order to complete the picture.

DISEASE CAUSES AND MECHANISMS

The root cause of PMS is almost always a disharmony between the liver and spleen. The liver becomes depressed, due to emotional stress and frustration, and the qi becomes stagnant. Worry, lack of exercise, overwork or improper diet cause the spleen to become vacuous and weak. Since, according to Chinese medicine, the liver controls the spleen, if the liver becomes depressed, this can cause or worsen spleen vacuity or weakness. Conversely, if the spleen is vacuous and weak, this may allow the liver to become even more depressed. Liver depression tends to arise or worsen during the premenstruum because the blood that was nourishing, softening and harmonising the liver is now being sent down to nourish the uterus. If there is not sufficient blood for both these purposes, the liver may not receive sufficient nourishment to perform its duty of controlling the coursing and discharge, i.e. the free flow, of the qi. If the liver does not course and discharge, the qi does not move freely and becomes stagnant.

The spleen is the root of qi and blood engenderment and transformation. If the spleen is vacuous and weak, then it may not engender and transform qi and blood sufficiently. If this happens, then, as we have just seen above, liver blood may become insufficient to allow the liver to perform its function of coursing and discharging the qi. On the other hand, if the spleen does not engender the qi sufficiently, the qi will lack its motivating force to move. Thus it is easy to see how closely these two viscera are related in terms of the free flow of the qi. The liver allows the qi to flow freely, but it is the spleen that is the ultimate source of the qi's power to move. Hence liver depression and spleen vacuity typically go hand in hand in clinical practice. In addition, we should remember that, because of their monthly loss of blood, the spleens of women must work harder at producing blood than the spleens of men. This also predisposes women in particular towards a spleen insufficiency. In my experience, liver depression spleen vacuity weakness is usually at the root of the disease mechanism behind PMS. I have never in 17 years of clinical practice seen a single case of PMS without at least some element of liver depression.

According to Chinese medical theory, if the liver becomes depressed and qi stagnant, this may eventually transform into pathological heat. Remember that the qi is inherently warm. If the qi becomes blocked and accumulates, backing up under pressure, all this depressed and stagnant yang qi will transform into what is called transformative or depressive heat. Over time, this pathological heat, being yang by nature, will consume and dry out kidney yin. Since, in Chinese medicine, yin is supposed to control yang, if kidney yin becomes vacuous and weak, liver yang may become hyperactive. Since fire burns upwards and the heart and lungs are located above the liver, this pathological heat may also accumulate in the heart and/or lungs, disturbing either of or both heart and lung function.

As mentioned above, since the spleen is the root of the engenderment and transformation of blood, if the spleen becomes weak, the blood may also become vacuous. Since some essence from the kidneys is required in order to make new blood, it is said in Chinese medicine that blood and essence share a common source. What this means in terms of disease mechanisms is that persistent blood vacuity may lead to insufficiency of kidney essence. This may aggravate any tendency to kidney yin vacuity that may already have been caused by damage due to chronic pathological heat.

As the spleen is also in charge of moving and transforming liquids, if the spleen becomes weak, water dampness may accumulate. Dampness, which is yin, being thick and turbid, may further block the free flow of qi, which is yang, aggravating liver depression. Dampness may also congeal and transform into phlegm. This phlegm impedes even further the free flow of qi and may lodge between the skin and flesh, in the channels and network vessels and in what are known as the clear orifices of the heart and head. Phlegm blocking the clear orifices of the heart gives rise to mental–emotional problems. The clear orifices of the head refer to the sensory organs of the eyes, ears, nose and mouth. If phlegm blocks any of these, then there will be some disturbance in the function of the associated sense. For example, if the orifices of the eyes are blocked by phlegm, then there will be problems with vision. If the orifices of the ears are blocked, there will be hearing problems.

In Chinese medicine, the functions of the spleen and stomach whilst in the process of digestion are likened to a pot on a stove and the subsequent production of qi and blood is likened to the distillation of alcohol. According to this metaphor, qi and blood are the distillation of foods and liquids cooked and transformed by the spleen and stomach. The source of heat for the spleen and stomach to perform their job is the kidney fire or kidney yang. If the spleen is chronically weak, the kidney yang may also become weak. Since kidney essence is the material basis of both kidney yin and yang, this process can be accelerated if there is long-term blood vacuity. On the other hand, long-lasting kidney yang vacuity and weakness will impair blood production as well. Thus, the correct functioning of the viscera and bowels are very dependent on each other and there is a close relationship between the liver and spleen and the spleen, stomach and kidneys.

This may seem quite complicated to someone new to Chinese medicine as it is a very complex system of thought and not just a primitive folk medicine. As we will see later, there are further mechanisms that may occur as a consequence of these main disease mechanisms. However, the mechanisms that we have just described are at the root of most premenstrual signs and symptoms. If you have an understanding of these mechanisms and a sound grasp of the basic theories of Chinese medicine discussed above, you can work out a rational explanation for any sign or symptom that a woman may experience before her menses.

TREATMENT ACCORDING TO PATTERN DISCRIMINATION

Fundamental to traditional Chinese medicine (TCM) is treatment based on what is known as 'pattern discrimination'. Modern Western medicine bases its treatment on a disease diagnosis. This means that two patients diagnosed as suffering from the same disease will get the same treatment. Whilst TCM does take the patient's disease diagnosis into account, the choice of treatment is not so much based on the disease diagnosis as it is on what is called the patient's pattern. This aspect of Chinese medicine makes it holistic, safe and effective.

In order to explain the difference between a disease and pattern, let us take the symptom of a headache as an example. All headaches by definition must involve some pain in the head. In modern Western medicine and other medical systems that prescribe primarily on the basis of a disease diagnosis, there is likely to be some sort of specific headache medication given. Headache sufferers could, however, be quite different – man or woman, young or old, overweight or thin, for example. The actual symptoms of the headache could also vary – the pain may be on the left or right side, it may be throbbing and continuous or sharp but intermittent, etc. One sufferer could also have the following symptoms: indigestion, a tendency to loose stools, cold feet, red eyes, a dry mouth and desire for cold drinks; another sufferer could have a wet, weeping, crusty skin rash with red borders, a tendency to hay fever, ringing in their ears and dizziness when they stand up. Whilst according to both Chinese medicine and modern Western medicine both people suffer from a headache, they also suffer from a whole host of other complaints and may have very different types of headaches, as well as very different constitutions, ages and sex. In Chinese medicine, the patient's pattern takes all of this information into account: the pattern tries to describe the totality of the person as a unique individual. Treatment is designed to rebalance that entire pattern of imbalance as well as address the major complaint, symptom or disease.

There is a saying in Chinese medicine: 'One disease, different treatments. Different diseases, same treatment.' In essence, this means that, in Chinese medicine, two patients with the same named disease diagnosis may receive different treatments if their Chinese medical patterns are different, while two patients diagnosed with different named diseases may receive the same treatment if their medical pattern is the same. The result is that each person is treated individually.

Since every patient gets an individually tailored treatment to restore balance, there are usually no side-effects. Side-effects come from forcing one part of the body to behave while causing an imbalance in some other part. The treatment may have been appropriate to relieve part of the problem but it does not take into account the whole. This is a little like robbing Peter to pay Paul. The fact that Chinese medicine takes so many aspects of a person into account in both diagnosis and treatment and looks at the body and mind as a single, unified whole means that a problem is treated without creating further imbalances.

Now we shall examine the major Chinese medical patterns at work in PMS.

Liver depression qi stagnation
Main symptoms
Premenstrual painful and swollen breasts, chest and rib-side pain, swollen lower abdomen, discomfort in the stomach and epigastrium (area above the stomach), diminished appetite, possible delayed menstruation where the amount could either be scanty or profuse, clots within the menstrual blood, menses unable to come easily, a normal or slightly dark tongue with thin, white fur and a bowstring, fine pulse[1].

Treatment principles
Correct the functioning of the liver and move the qi, rectify the blood and regulate the menses.

---

[1] Taking the pulse forms an important part of Chinese medical diagnosis. There are six different pulse positions on the radial artery of each wrist, giving information about the viscera, bowels and channels. There are 28 different types of pulse quality according to classic Chinese medicine, including bowstring, fine, deep, empty, etc.

Spleen–kidney yang vacuity

Main symptoms

Oedema (fluid retention) either before or after the menses, dizziness, lumbar pain and fatigue in the limbs, reduced appetite, loose stools or diarrhoea before the menses, stomach and epigastric distension and fullness, lack of warmth in the hands and feet, a pale facial complexion, menses scanty in amount, a fat tongue with thin, white or slimy, white fur and a deep, fine, weak pulse.

In clinical practice, this pattern never presents in this simple, discrete manner in PMS. Spleen qi and kidney yang vacuity do however typically complicate most cases of PMS in women in their late 30s and 40s. According to my clinical experience, there will also be liver depression present in all cases. I therefore choose a prescription that remedies spleen vacuity and modify it for liver depression; if liver depression is the predominant pattern, I choose a formula for liver depression and modify it for spleen and kidney vacuity.

Treatment principles

Warm the kidneys, fortify the spleen and promote the flow of water within the body.

Heart–spleen dual vacuity

Main symptoms

Heart palpitations either before or after the menses, loss of sleep, lassitude of the spirit (apathy), lack of strength, a slightly puffy face, profuse or scanty menses that are pale in colour, a pale tongue with thin, white fur and a soggy, small or fine, weak pulse.

Heart–spleen dual vacuity means heart blood vacuity and spleen qi vacuity. If heart blood vacuity is more prominent, the amount of menstrual blood is scanty. If spleen qi vacuity is more prominent, the amount of discharge is profuse. In both cases, the colour of the menstrual blood tends to be pale. If the spleen is vacuous and, therefore, also damp, the pulse will be soggy. If blood is vacuous, the pulse will be fine. As with the above pattern, this one also is rarely, if ever, seen in its simple, discrete form in clinical practice. Commonly, if there is heart blood vacuity, this merely complicates liver depression and spleen vacuity. If the liver depression is secondary in importance, then I would choose a main guiding formula which primarily supplements and nourishes the heart and spleen, modifying it for liver depression. If liver depression is primary, then I would modify a formula suitable to treat that pattern.

Treatment principles
Supplement and nourish the heart, spleen, qi and blood.

Kidney vacuity liver effulgence
Main symptoms
Menstruation either early or late, lumbar pain, numb hands and feet, one-sided headache, tinnitus, blurred vision, distension and pain that feels as if it stretches from the lower abdomen to the chest and breasts, frequent, short urination, menstruation that is brief and profuse, tongue coating that is shiny and peeled, a fat tongue with purple edges and a deep, small, bowstring pulse.

Although not stated in the Chinese title of this pattern, liver qi depression and stagnation are a part of this scenario. This is evidenced by the feeling of lower abdominal distension and pain reaching to the chest and breasts and also by the bowstring pulse. In this case, liver depression transforms into fire and causes the blood to move recklessly leading to a profuse menstrual flow. Since liver blood is relatively vacuous or empty, the length of the menses is short.

Treatment principles
Boost the kidneys and regulate the liver.

THE REAL DEAL

In clinical practice it is rare to encounter one of the patterns outlined above in isolation. Since all the viscera and bowels are interconnected and related, the impaired functioning of one impacts on the others. So it is more usual to see combinations of the above patterns and their related disease mechanisms or progressions. In trying to identify all the mechanisms I have encountered in women with PMS, I have come up with the following list:

Liver depression qi stagnation
Depressive heat
Spleen qi vacuity
Spleen dampness
Liver blood vacuity
Kidney yin vacuity
Spleen–kidney yang vacuity
Replete (excessive) heat in the heart, lungs and/or stomach
Vacuity heat in the heart, lungs and/or stomach (due to
    hyperactive yang)
Heart qi and/or blood vacuity
Liver yang hyperactivity
Liver fire flaring above
Stirring of liver wind
Food stagnation
Phlegm confounding (blocking) the orifices
Phlegm fire
Damp heat accumulating below
Blood stasis
External invasion (of pathogens)
Retained evils or deep-lying warm evils (pathogens lying
    latent in the body)

In all cases of PMS, liver qi plays a central role. This is because the premenstruum and the menstrual movement are concerned with yang reaching its maximum and transforming into yin (just as ovulation concerns yin reaching its maximum and transforming into yang). Such transformation can only proceed correctly if the qi mechanism is free-flowing and uninhibited. The qi mechanism's free and uninhibited flow is dependent on the liver's coursing and discharge. This means liver depression qi stagnation is at the heart of every woman's PMS.

Since there are complex relationships between the liver and all the other viscera and bowels of Chinese medicine, and also between the qi, blood, fluids and essence, liver depression qi stagnation may be complicated or evolve into a number of other patterns. In clinical practice, it is essential to identify the main disease mechanism currently at work and choose a guiding formula or treatment based on rebalancing this imbalance. This guiding formula is then modified to address the other associated disease mechanisms, signs and symptoms. Should the symptoms disappear after treating a fundamental or basic disease mechanism, then it is not necessary to address specifically any secondary or dependent disease mechanisms.

If you can understand the interrelationships between the above 20 mechanisms, then you can diagnose and understand the premenstrual symptoms of any woman. These 20 mechanisms or patterns have an underlying logic; they are not a random collection.

We have already discussed the relationships between the first seven mechanisms above. If liver depression transforms into depressive heat, this heat may flow upwards and harass the heart, lungs and/or stomach. On the other hand, if liver blood–kidney vacuity gives rise to vacuity heat, this vacuity heat could flow upwards to harass the heart, lungs and/or stomach and damage their yin fluids. Since both heart qi and blood have their source in the spleen's engenderment and transformation of food and drink, if the spleen is vacuous and weak, this may easily give rise to either heart blood or heart qi vacuity. If depressive heat damages yin, yang will become effulgent and give rise to liver yang hyperactivity. If such liver yang hyperactivity becomes even worse, it may become liver fire (pathogens created within the body) flaring above, while liver fire and/or liver blood vacuity may engender internal stirring of liver wind (an unseen pathogen that has invaded the liver's defences).

In the Yuan dynasty (1280–1368 AD), Zhu Dan-xi, one of the four great masters of medicine of his time, explained that if qi becomes stagnant and the spleen becomes weak this can easily result in food stagnation. Food stagnation means food sits in the stomach undigested. Such food stagnation may also transform depressive heat. If dampness due to the spleen not moving and transporting fluids continues to gather, it may congeal into phlegm. However, phlegm may also be due to intense heat steaming and fuming the fluids, congealing them into phlegm (like cooking a pudding on top of a stove). In both cases, phlegm, being a yin depression, obstructs the free and uninhibited flow of qi and blood. It may gather and cause obstruction in the area between the skin and muscles or flesh, within the viscera and bowels and within the channels and network vessels. It may also confound and block the clear (sensory) orifices, i.e. the nose, ears, eyes and mouth, or the orifices of the heart. If the clear orifices are blocked, there will be a reduction or loss of sensual acuity of the associated orifice. If the orifices of the heart are confounded, there will be disturbed or diminished mental–emotional function.

Dampness, which is heavy and turbid, tends to percolate and pour downwards. It obstructs the free flow of qi, blood and fluids. If damp depression gives rise to depressive heat, then dampness may become damp heat. It is also possible for liver depression transformative heat to stew the juices and give rise to damp heat. If qi stagnation means the blood doesn't move, the blood will stop and become static. So, if the liver depression is severe and persistent enough, it may give rise to blood stasis. Static blood is like silt in the blood vessels and, like silt that blocks a river, it may eventually clog and obstruct the flow of blood in the affected area. Blood stasis is mainly associated with the symptom of pain, such as menstrual or premenstrual lower abdominal pain, premenstrual breast pain, headache or other relatively severe aches and pains. The pain resulting from blood stasis tends to be fixed in location and sharp or piercing in nature.

As the spleen and stomach form the source of the defensive qi, if the spleen becomes premenstrually vacuous and weak, there may be a defensive qi vacuity. Such a pre-menstrual defensive qi vacuity is often aggravated by blood vacuity. The blood is sent down to the uterus before menstruation, leaving the upper body relatively empty and insufficient of blood, especially in women whose blood production tends to be poor. The blood and the constructive qi are closely related. So a blood and constructive qi vacuity in the upper body leads to a disharmony between the defensive and constructive qi. This results in external pathogens easily being able to take advantage of this vacuity and enter the body, leading to recurrent colds or flu before the menses.

It is also possible that either 'retained evils' or 'deep-lying warm evils' may become active during the premenstruum. Retained evils are pathogens that have invaded the body at some previous time. For some reason, perhaps due to incomplete recovery from an illness or incorrect treatment at the time of the illness, these pathogens have not all been eliminated from the body. They may linger, latent, in the body. Given the appropriate internal environment, they may become active again. Hidden or deep-lying warm evils are warm or damp heat pathogens that enter the body but do not cause disease at that time. Rather, they lie latent until the internal conditions in the body are conducive to their being able to thrive and become active. The premenstrual conditions that include the presence of dampness, depressive heat and a lack of righteous qi affecting the spleen and/or kidneys create the ideal environment for retained or deep-lying warm evils to thrive. This helps explain premenstrual outbreaks of herpes and cold sores.

All signs and symptoms of PMS can be diagnosed and treated according to Chinese medicine based on various combinations of the above disease mechanisms and patterns. In order to make this work, you must have a firm grasp of the defining or main symptoms of each pattern. Since Chinese medicine takes years of study, this is obviously not something a layperson could do. However, if you can identify or have a general idea of your predominant pattern, there is a lot you can do for yourself. Hopefully, some of the signs and symptoms listed in the main patterns discussed earlier will be familiar and you may be able to recognise them in yourself. If so, see which pattern includes the majority of your signs and symptoms as this is probably the main pattern or disease mechanism accounting for your PMS. Even if you only address the main pattern and miss some of the minor complications, you should experience some relief of your symptoms. Since all woman with PMS will have liver depression qi stagnation, as either the main pattern or a secondary mechanism, following the dietary, exercise and lifestyle recommendations for this pattern will be helpful to everyone.

HOW THE SYSTEM WORKS IN REAL LIFE

As we have discussed, if you are able to identify from a Chinese medical perspective which patterns and disease mechanisms are occurring, your PMS can be very effectively treated. We shall now examine how this system works in real life.

DENISE'S CASE

Take Denise, whom I introduced at the beginning of this book. Each month she is tired, irritable and upset before her period. Not only does she get angry for little or no reason, but she tends to cry at the drop of a hat. Her periods tend to be late, coming anywhere between 33–45 days apart. Before her menses start, she has lower abdominal bloating and cramping for a couple of days. During the first few hours of her period, she has more severe cramps, which are relieved by rubbing, applying heat, or, if she can get herself to do it, some light exercise. Her breasts become sore and distended before her menses, with her nipples becoming especially sensitive and having a sore or inflamed feeling. Denise tends to be constipated right up until the day her menses start and then she has loose stools for a day. If she eats a large meal, her abdomen becomes bloated and it feels as if her food is just sitting in her stomach all day. Nevertheless, she finds that her appetite is increased premenstrually, and she particularly craves sweets and carbohydrates. To add insult to injury, a few days before her period, Denise gets two or three fairly large, red spots at the corners of her mouth. Her tongue is a normal colour with a slightly yellow coating; it is a little swollen and one can see the indentations of her teeth along its edges.

There is a bitter taste in her mouth when Denise wakes up in the morning. Her pulse is bowstring, overall. However, her right pulse in the position which corresponds to the spleen and stomach is fine, floating and bowstring.

Analysis of Denise's symptoms according to TCM

In Chinese medicine, anger is the emotion associated with the liver. So Denise's problem of irritability and becoming upset easily would immediately lead us to suspect that liver depression qi stagnation is playing a part in her PMS. We know that liver depression typically gets worse during the premenstruum due to the collection of blood in the uterus, which leaves the liver 'high and dry'. Denise is not just irritable, she also tends to cry at little things which, at other times of the month, would not provoke such a tearful reaction. Grief and melancholy are the emotions associated with the lungs in Chinese medicine, while tears are the fluid associated with the liver ('the liver opens into the portals of the eyes'). This crying for little reason is typically due to some sort of pathological relationship between the liver and lungs. Pathological heat tends to force body fluids to 'run recklessly outside of the body'. So, it may be due to pathological heat in the lungs that Denise cries so easily.

As we have already discussed, if liver depression continues for a long period of time, it can easily transform into depressive heat. Heat, as it is yang in nature, has an innate tendency to travel upwards. Remember, the lungs are referred to as 'the florid canopy' meaning that the lungs are the capstone of the other viscera and bowels and so heat wafting upwards from the liver below often accumulates and lodges in the lungs. This is corroborated by the fact that Denise has a bitter taste in her mouth in the morning. This bitter taste is due to bile which, like tears, is another of the body's fluids associated with the liver. If there is depressive heat in the liver, this heat may force bile to flow recklessly upwards to the mouth and result in a bitter taste.

We also know that Denise experiences premenstrual breast distension and soreness. Distension is categorised as qi stagnation and accumulation, and we have already seen that the qi of the chest and breasts has a special relationship with the liver. If liver qi becomes depressed and stagnant and then counterflows horizontally, it may accumulate in the breasts and chest. The fact that this liver qi has transformed into depressive heat is indicated by Denise's nipples becoming sore and inflamed premenstrually (the liver channel 'homes' to the nipples). This means that a feeling of heat in the nipples suggests depressive liver heat. Denise's spots are red, indicating the presence of heat according to Chinese medicine. Spots and pimples are skin lesions and as we saw in the earlier table the lungs govern the skin and body hair, so red skin lesions often suggest heat in the lungs. The presence of heat in the lungs is corroborated by the tendency to cry discussed above. The location of the spots under the corners of the mouth suggest that this heat is also affecting the stomach, as this area of the face is traversed by the stomach channel. Denise's increased appetite is another possible symptom of stomach heat and this is corroborated by the slightly yellowish tongue coating, which also indicates that heat has affected the stomach. This is because the tongue coating is taken as an indication of the stomach qi, and yellow as opposed to white fur indicates heat.

The other signs and symptoms that add up to liver depression qi stagnation according to the principles of Chinese medicine include the premenstrual lower abdomen distension and cramping and the menstrual cramps on the first day of the period that are relieved by massage, warmth and exercise. In Chinese medicine, it is said: 'If there is pain, there is no free flow. If there is free flow, there is no pain.'

Since there is premenstrual and menstrual cramping, we know that the flow of qi and blood is not free and easy. Massage, warmth and exercise all help to mobilise the qi and blood and promote free flow. So Denise's dysmenorrhoea (painful menstruation) also corroborates a Chinese pattern discrimination of liver depression qi stagnation. The fact that Denise's periods are always coming late and at irregular intervals suggests that depressed qi is not allowing the blood to flow freely from the body. Finally, a bowstring pulse is 'the pulse of the liver' and is the definitive pulse image denoting liver depression and constraint.

Now let's look at Denise's fatigue and tiredness. We already know that the spleen is the root of qi and blood production and fatigue is always a symptom of qi vacuity or weakness. The fact that the spleen qi in particular is weak and insufficient is corroborated first by the fact that Denise gets bloated after heavy meals. It is the spleen's job to 'disperse and transform' the digestate and, if it is weak, it cannot do this, so resulting in indigestion. Secondly, Denise's tongue is swollen and has the indentations of her teeth along its edges. The spleen is responsible for moving and transforming body fluids. If the spleen qi is weak, these body fluids accumulate and transform into dampness and produce a swollen, oedematous tongue. Third, Denise's cravings for sweets and carbohydrates (which are metabolised into sugar) are an indication of spleen vacuity. Sweetness 'gathers' in the spleen and sweet is a 'supplementing' flavour, engendering both more qi and more fluids. A little sweet flavour supplements the spleen qi, but too much actually damages the spleen further and leads to the formation of internal dampness. Lastly, the floating, fine pulse in the middle position on the right wrist corresponding to the spleen also indicates spleen vacuity and dampness.

The fact that Denise is constipated premenstrually and then has loose stools on day one of her period shows that liver depression qi stagnation is affecting her spleen function. The Chinese medical term for this is that the liver is 'assailing' the spleen. Premenstrually, liver depression fails to 'course and discharge' and so the stools are not discharged and precipitated. On the first day of the period, since blood has started to be lost, the spleen becomes even weaker than it was premenstrually. This results in loose stools since spleen vacuity is one of the leading causes of diarrhoea. The fact that the liver is assailing or invading the spleen is corroborated by the bowstring quality of the right middle pulse position as well as its being floating and fine.

In summary, the practitioner of Chinese medicine analyses Denise's PMS and comes to the conclusion that the disease mechanisms involved are a combination of three factors: liver depression transforming into heat; depressive heat counterflowing upwards and accumulating in the stomach and lungs; and spleen vacuity, possibly with some dampness.

Treatment of Denise's PMS with Chinese medicine

Once the practitioner has diagnosed the patient's pattern discrimination, the next step is to formulate the treatment principles necessary to correct the imbalance implied by this pattern discrimination. If liver depression qi stagnation is the main or leading pattern, then the first treatment principles are to course the liver and rectify the qi. These are the treatment principles for correcting liver depression qi stagnation. To course the liver means to promote the liver's coursing and discharge, or spreading, of the qi freely and easily throughout the body. Rectifying the qi means to make the qi move and, more than that, move in the right directions. If the second element in the pattern discrimination is depressive heat in the stomach and lungs, then the second set of principles is to clear heat and resolve depression from those organs. Finally, if the third element in the pattern discrimination is spleen vacuity with possible dampness, then the necessary treatment principles for rebalancing this are to fortify (strengthen) the spleen and supplement the qi and possibly to eliminate dampness.

Once the practitioner has diagnosed the patterns and stated the treatment principles, then anything that works to accomplish these principles will be beneficial for the patient. Various treatment modalities are open to the practitioner, the main two being acupuncture (see page 82) and herbal medicine (see page 69). They can also significantly help the patient with appropriate dietary and lifestyle advice and recommendations.

In China the most popular treatment modality is herbal medicine, whilst in the UK it is more likely to be acupuncture as there are far fewer trained herbalists here. Both treatments are extremely effective for PMS and may be used alone or in combination with each other.

Let's look at Denise and her PMS, and how a Chinese herbal prescription could help. In her case the liver is depressed and the spleen is weak, which means there is a disharmony between the liver and spleen. There is yet another disharmony between the spleen, which is weak, and the stomach, which is hot. So the Chinese herbalist would start by choosing a formula from the 'harmonising' category of Chinese medicinal formulae. They would look for a harmonising formula that courses the liver and rectifies the qi, clears heat in the stomach and lungs, fortifies the spleen and supplements the qi.

Of the various harmonising formulae, there is a well-known one that does exactly these things. It is called *Xiao Chai Hu Tang* (Minor Bupleurum Decoction). Let's look at its ingredients and see how they work. This formula is composed of:

Radix Bupleuri *(Chai Hu)*
Radix Panacis Ginseng *(Ren Shen)*
Rhizoma Pinelliae Ternatae *(Ban Xia)*
Radix Scutellariae Baicalensis *(Huang Qin)*
Mix-fried Radix Glycyrrhizae *(Gan Cao)*
Fructus Zizyphi Jujubae *(Da Zao)*
Uncooked Rhizoma Zingiberis *(Sheng Jiang)*

Radix Bupleuri courses the liver and rectifies the qi. It is the single most commonly used Chinese medicinal for remedying liver depression qi stagnation. Radix Panacis Ginseng is the most well-known spleen-fortifying qi supplement in Chinese medicine. However, Ginseng also quiets the spirit. Rhizoma Pinelliae Ternatae helps Bupleurum regulate the qi and move downwards any upward counterflow. At the same time, it helps Ginseng to fortify the spleen. If there is any dampness, Pinellia would also transform dampness or phlegm. Radix Scutellariae Baicalensis clears heat specifically from the liver, stomach and lungs, the three organs that have accumulated depressive heat in this case. Mix-fried Radix Glycyrrhizae (liquorice) helps Ginseng and Pinellia fortify the spleen and supplement the qi. Liquorice, in particular, supplements the spleen and heart qi. Liquorice also moderates harsh actions of any of the medicinals in this formula and helps the other medicinals to act in a concerted and harmonious way. Fructus Zizyphi Jujubae (red dates) also fortifies the spleen and supplements the qi, thus aiding the other spleen supplements in this formula. Red dates also nourish the heart blood and, like Ginseng, help to calm the heart spirit. Uncooked Rhizoma Zingiberis (ginger) promotes the flow of qi. It also harmonises the stomach and helps eliminate dampness as well as helping liquorice to harmonise and moderate all the other ingredients.

We can see that the ingredients in this formula embody and carry out very precisely and specifically the treatment principles necessary for rebalancing Denise's condition. In fact, this formula is the most frequently prescribed Chinese medicinal formula in the world. It is used to treat a very wide range of diseases in patients presenting with a pattern of liver depression and spleen vacuity with heat in either the liver, stomach or lungs. This formula is not used exclusively to treat PMS but may be used to treat everything from chronic bronchitis, nausea and diarrhoea to chronic tonsillitis, chronic hepatitis and a whole host of gynaecological complaints. Its choice has little to do with Western disease diagnosis and everything to do with Chinese pattern discrimination.

To make this formula even more effective, the Chinese herbalist will frequently further modify it by taking out one or more of the ingredients and adding others in order to tailor it to the patient's exact configuration of signs and symptoms. Since Denise's case is one of PMS due primarily to aggravation of premenstrual liver depression, in turn due to blood collecting in the uterus and leaving the liver 'high and dry', I would add Radix Angelicae Sinensis *(Dang Gui)* and Radix Albus Paeoniae Lactiflorae *(Bai Shao)* to the basic formula. These two medicinals both nourish the blood and soften and harmonise the liver. Since they also quicken the blood, they will also ease Denise's period pains. If the signs and symptoms of spleen vacuity and dampness are more pronounced, then I might add two more medicinals for fortifying the spleen and eliminating dampness: Rhizoma Atractylodis Macrocephalae *(Bai Zhu)* and Sclerotium Poriae Cocos *(Fu Ling)*. If breast distension is more pronounced, I might add a couple more ingredients for rectifying or regulating the qi in the chest and breasts, such as Rhizoma Cyperi Rotundi *(Xiang Fu)* and Radix Linderae Strychnofoliae *(Wu Yao)*. These should also help eliminate the period pain. If depressive heat is more pronounced, then I might add one or more medicinals for clearing heat, such as Fructus Gardeniae Jasminoidis *(Shan Zhi Zi)*, Rhizoma Coptidis Chinensis *(Huang Lian)*, or Herba Taraxaci Mongolici Cum Radice *(Pu Gong Ying)*. This last ingredient would be a good choice because Herba Taraxaci Mongolici Cum Radice (dandelion) not only clears heat, it courses the liver qi and promotes the flow of qi specifically in the breasts. Whenever possible, we try to use the least number of ingredients to achieve the maximum effect.

Usually, a formula such as this when used to treat PMS would be started as soon as the symptoms manifested each month and would be continued through the first day of the onset of the menses. The ingredients in this formula may be dispensed in bulk and then brewed as a 'tea' by the patient or may be taken as a dried, powdered extract. Many standard formulae also come in pill form. However, these cannot be modified. If their ingredients match the individual patient's requirements, then they work well, but if the formula needs modification, then teas or powders whose individual ingredients can be added and subtracted are more appropriate.

In exactly the same way, i.e. by looking at Denise's signs and symptoms and identifying any underlying imbalances, an acupuncture treatment could be devised. The practitioner could also create an accompanying dietary and lifestyle plan. We will discuss each of these later on in the book. In a woman of Denise's age with her Chinese pattern discrimination, either Chinese herbal medicine alone, acupuncture alone, or a combination of the two supported by the proper diet and lifestyle would usually eliminate or at the very least drastically diminish her PMS within three months, meaning three menstrual cycles.

CHINESE HERBAL MEDICINE AND PMS

As we have seen from Denise's case, there is no one specific herb or even formula to treat the symptoms of PMS. Chinese herbal medicine is given based on the diagnosis of a pattern discrimination. PMS is in itself too broad a category for there to be a single prescription for its treatment. In fact it can be detrimental to your health and well-being if you use the wrong herbs. Take ginseng for example: if a woman has PMS and none of her symptoms are due to spleen qi vacuity, then ginseng is not going to help her. If her pattern is liver depression transforming into heat or ascendant hyperactivity of liver yang, she may very well find herself having more headaches, more irritability, more red, painful eyes and more dizziness, if she takes sufficient ginseng over a period of time. Since this woman's qi is depressed, adding more qi (which is to a certain extent the effect of taking ginseng) to qi that is already not flowing freely only adds to this depression which, under pressure, transforms into heat and vents itself upwards to harass the head. On the other hand, if a woman with PMS does display signs and symptoms of spleen qi vacuity, then the right amount of ginseng would be very beneficial.

In a similar way, if a woman with PMS also manifests the signs and symptoms of blood vacuity or blood stasis, then taking *Dang Gui* will probably help relieve some of her symptoms. *Dang Gui* nourishes and quickens the blood. By nourishing the blood, it softens and harmonises the liver. This does not address liver depression completely and directly, but it does help. By quickening the blood, *Dang Gui* does help to treat pain due to blood stasis, especially blood stasis period pain. If, however, a woman does not have much blood vacuity or blood stasis, then *Dang Gui* will not have much effect on her PMS.

Since PMS is a combination of different Chinese patterns and disease mechanisms, Chinese herbal medicine would not treat it with a single herb. Chinese herbal medicine is based on rebalancing patterns, and patterns in real-life patients almost always have more than a single element. This is why herbal formulae in Chinese medicine have many ingredients, usually up to 18 or more. A practitioner of Chinese herbal medicine would be able to identify the patient's most likely pattern discrimination and what the most likely signs and symptoms were by looking at a herbal prescription. Each herbal formula is carefully crafted to deal with the patient on an individual basis, taking into account all aspects of their body and mind.

GETTING THE RIGHT HERBAL MEDICINE TREATMENT FOR YOURSELF

Chinese herbal medicine requires a high level of study and skill and I strongly recommend that you seek professional advice. As well as the signs and symptoms of the illness, the practitioner will take into account additional information such as tongue and pulse diagnosis. These skills require experience and training that are beyond the scope of this book. As a layperson it is unlikely that you will be able to obtain Chinese herbs without a prescription from a qualified practitioner, as reputable suppliers don't sell directly to the public. Details of how to find a properly qualified practitioner will be given later (see pages 145–48). Chinese herbal medicine is very powerful and only really safe if properly and correctly prescribed. After all, if a herb is strong enough to heal an imbalance, it is also strong enough to create an imbalance if given in the wrong dose or incorrectly prescribed.

CHINESE PATENT MEDICINES

The remainder of this chapter will focus on what are commonly known as Chinese patent herbal remedies or 'patents'. These are herbal remedies that have been used for many years, often centuries, and therefore have a tried and tested track record for treating illness. In some countries these may be available in a health shop or specialist Chinese herb shop, but I strongly recommend that you do not take them unsupervised. I have included them here as they demonstrate how Chinese herbal medicine treats PMS; in fact, even an individually tailored herbal formula will often be based on one of the formulae here.

Earlier, I gave the signs and symptoms of four of the key patterns associated with most women's PMS. These are:

Liver depression qi stagnation
Spleen–kidney yang vacuity
Heart–spleen dual vacuity
Kidney vacuity liver effulgence

If you are able to identify your main pattern from one of these, then it is likely that the relevant Chinese patent could be beneficial.

Xiao Yao Wan (also spelt *Hsiao Yao Wan)*
Xiao Yao Wan is one of the most common Chinese herbal formulae prescribed to women suffering from PMS. Its Chinese name has been translated as Free and Easy Pills, Rambling Pills, Relaxed Wanderer Pills and several other versions of this same idea of promoting a freer and smoother, more relaxed flow. As a patent medicine, this formula comes as pills and there are both Chinese and American versions of this formula available. The ingredients in this formula are:

Radix Bupleuri *(Chai Hu)*
Radix Angelicae Sinensis *(Dang Gui)*
Radix Albus Paeoniae Lactiflorae *(Bai Shao)*
Rhizoma Atractylodis Macrocephalae *(Bai Zhu)*
Sclerotium Poriae Cocos *(Fu Ling)*
Mix-fried Radix Glycyrrhizae *(Gan Cao)*
Herba Menthae Haplocalycis *(Bo He)*
Uncooked Rhizoma Zingiberis *(Sheng Jiang)*

This formula treats the pattern of liver depression qi stagnation complicated by blood vacuity and spleen weakness with possible dampness as well. Bupleurum courses the liver and rectifies the qi. It is aided in this by Herba Menthae Haplocalycis (peppermint). *Dang Gui* and Radix Albus Paeoniae Lactilforae (white peony) nourish the blood and soften and harmonise the liver. Rhizoma Atractylodis Macrocephalae and Sclerotium Poriae Cocos fortify the spleen and eliminate dampness. Mix-fried Glycyrrhiza (liquorice) aid these two in fortifying the spleen and supplementing the liver, while uncooked Zingiber (ginger) aids in both promoting and regulating the qi flow and eliminating dampness.

When PMS presents with the signs and symptoms of liver depression and spleen vacuity, you can try taking this formula as soon as any symptoms appear and continue taking it throughout the first day of menstruation. If, after taking these pills at the dose recommended on the packaging, you notice any side-effects, then stop immediately and seek professional advice. Side-effects from this formula might include nervousness, irritability, a dry mouth, increased thirst and red, dry eyes. Such side-effects would suggest that this formula is not right for you, at least without some modification. Although it may be doing you some good, it is also causing some harm. Remember, Chinese medicine is meant to cure without side-effects and as long as the prescription matches one's pattern there should not be any.

Dan Zhi Xiao Yao Wan

Dan Zhi Xiao Yao Wan or Moutan and Gardenia Rambling Pills is a modification of the previous formula that also comes as a patent medicine in the form of pills. It is meant to treat the pattern of liver depression transforming into heat with spleen vacuity and possible blood vacuity and/or dampness. The ingredients in this formula are the same as before except that two other herbs are added:

Cortex Radicis Moutan *(Dan Pi)*
Fructus Gardeniae Jasminoidis *(Shan Zhi Zi)*

These two ingredients clear heat and resolve depression. In addition, Cortex Radicis Moutan quickens the blood and dispels stasis and is good at clearing heat, specifically from the blood. Some practitioners suggest leaving out uncooked Zingiber and Mentha, while others leave them in.

Basically, the signs and symptoms of the pattern for which this formula is designed are the same as those for *Xiao Yao Wan* (see page 71) plus signs and symptoms of depressive heat. These might include a reddish tongue with slightly yellow fur, a bowstring and rapid pulse, a bitter taste in the mouth and increased irritability.

Shu Gan Wan (also spelt Shu Kan Wan)

Shu Gan Wan means Soothe the Liver Pills. This Chinese patent medicine is made up almost entirely of liver-coursing and qi-rectifying medicinals. Unlike *Xiao Yao Wan* (see page 71), it does not nourish the blood or supplement the spleen. Its ingredients are:

Fructus Meliae Toosendan *(Chuan Lian Zi)*
Rhizoma Curcumae Longae *(Jiang Huang)*
Lignum Aquilariae Agallochae *(Chen Xiang)*
Rhizoma Corydalis Yanhusuo *(Yan Hu Suo)*
Radix Auklandiae Lappae *(Mu Xiang)*
Semen Alpiniae Katsumadai *(Dou Kou)*
Radix Albus Paeoniae Lactiflorae *(Bai Shao)*
Sclerotium Poriae Cocos *(Fu Ling)*
Fructus Citri Aurantii *(Zhi Ke)*
Pericarpium Citri Reticulatae *(Chen Pi)*
Fructus Amomi *(Sha Ren)*
Cortex Magnoliae Officinalis *(Hou Po)*

This formula can be taken by itself when PMS really only consists of breast and abdominal distension and cramping. However, you can take these pills along with *Xiao Yao Wan* if there is liver depression and spleen and/or blood vacuity with more pronounced breast and/or abdominal distension and menstrual cramps. If taking these pills causes feelings of dryness or heat internally, or increased irritability, their dosage should be reduced or they should be stopped.

Xiang Sha Liu Jun Wan
The name of these pills translates as Auklandia and Amomum Six Gentlemen Pills. Sometimes they are referred to as Aplotaxis-Amomum Pills. This formula treats the pattern of pronounced spleen vacuity with elements of dampness and a little qi stagnation. Since the overwhelming majority of episodes of PMS include liver depression qi stagnation, these pills can be taken along with *Xiao Yao Wan* (see page 71) in those cases where spleen vacuity is more severe. These pills are especially good for treating poor appetite, nausea, abdominal bloating after meals and loose stools due to spleen vacuity and dampness. Their ingredients include:

Radix Codonopsitis Pilosulae *(Dang Shen)*
Rhizoma Atractylodis Macrocephalae *(Bai Zhu)*
Sclerotium Poriae Cocos *(Fu Ling)*
Rhizoma Pinelliae Ternatae *(Ban Xia)*
Mix-fried Radix Glycyrrhizae *(Gan Cao)*
Pericarpium Citri Reticulatae *(Chen Pi)*
Radix Auklandiae Lappae *(Mu Xiang)*
Fructus Amomi *(Sha Ren)*

Do not take these pills, however, if there is burning around the anus with bowel movements or there is diarrhoea with dark-coloured, foul-smelling, explosive stools.

Bu Zhong Yi Qi Wan

Bu Zhong Yi Qi Wan means Supplement the Centre and Boost the Qi Pills. This formula treats the pattern of central qi vacuity or central qi fall. The central qi is another name for the spleen and stomach qi. This formula is especially good for treating spleen vacuity weakness that manifests not so much as digestive complaints and diarrhoea but as more pronounced fatigue and orthostatic hypotension (dizziness on standing up). The ingredients in this formula are:

Radix Astaragli Membranacei *(Huang Qi)*
Radix Codonopsitis Pilosulae *(Dang Shen)*
Rhizoma Atractylodis Macrocephalae *(Bai Zhu)*
Mix-fried Radix Glycyrrhizae *(Gan Cao)*
Radix Angelicae Sinensis *(Dang Gui)*
Radix Bupleuri *(Chai Hu)*
Rhizoma Cimicifugae *(Sheng Ma)*
Pericarpium Citri Reticulatae *(Chen Pi)*
Fructus Zizyphi Jujubae *(Da Zao)*
Uncooked Rhizoma Zingiberis *(Sheng Jiang)*

This is actually a very sophisticated formula and it has a very wide range of applications. Since it includes Bupleurum and Angelica *(Dang Gui)*, it courses the liver and rectifies the qi as well as nourishing the blood and softening the liver. It can be added to *Xiao Yao Wan* (see page 71) when spleen vacuity causing fatigue is more pronounced. Since spleen vacuity typically does become more pronounced after the age of 35, these pills are often the guiding prescription or are combined with other formulae.

Ba Zhen Wan

Ba Zhen Wan literally means Eight Pearls Pills. However, these are also often marketed under the name Women's Precious Pills. The eight pearls refer to the four ingredients that supplement the qi and four ingredients that nourish the blood. These pills can be combined with *Xiao Yao Wan* (see page 71) when there is liver depression complicated by more serious spleen qi and liver blood vacuity. Their ingredients are:

Radix Codonopsitis Pilosulae *(Dang Shen)*
Rhizoma Atractylodis Macrocephalae *(Bai Zhu)*
Sclerotium Poriae Cocos *(Fu Ling)*
Mix-fried Radix Glycyrrhizae *(Gan Cao)*
Radix Angelicae Sinensis *(Dang Gui)*
Radix Albus Paeoniae Lactiflorae *(Bai Shao)*
Cooked Radix Rehmanniae *(Shu Di)*
Radix Ligustici Wallichii *(Chuan Xiong)*

Shi Quan Da Bu Wan

The name of these pills translates as Ten (Ingredients) Completely and Greatly Supplementing Pills. Their ingredients are the same as *Ba Zhen Wan* (above) plus:

Cortex Cinnamomi Cassiae *(Rou Gui)*
Radix Astragali Membranacei *(Huang Qi)*

Some practitioners feel that these extra two ingredients help the body generate new qi and blood more rapidly. Therefore, it can be added to *Xiao Yao Wan* (see page 71) for the same reasons as *Ba Zhen Wan*. However, because Cortex Cinnamomi Cassiae (cinnamon bark) is hot, it should not be used if there is depressive heat. It would not usually be combined with *Dan Zhi Xiao Yao Wan* (see page 73).

Tabellae Suan Zao Ren Tang

This is a tablet version of the formula *Suan Zao Ren Tang* (Zizyphus Seed Decoction). It treats insomnia and mental unrest due to liver blood vacuity. It can, therefore, be combined with *Xiao Yao Wan* (see page 71) when liver blood vacuity is more severe and manifests primarily as insomnia. Its ingredients are:

Semen Zizyphi Spinosae *(Suan Zao Ren)*
Sclerotium Poriae Cocos *(Fu Ling)*
Radix Ligustici Wallichii *(Chuan Xiong)*
Rhizoma Anemarrhenae Aspheloidis *(Zhi Mu)*
Mix-fried Radix Glycyrrhizae *(Gan Cao)*

Gui Pi Wan (also spelt *Kuei Pi Wan)*

Gui means to return or restore, *pi* means the spleen and *wan* means pills. So the name of these pills translates as Restore the Spleen Pills. However, these pills not only supplement the spleen qi but also nourish heart blood and calm the heart spirit. This is the textbook guiding formula for the pattern of heart–spleen dual vacuity when there are symptoms of spleen qi vacuity, such as fatigue, poor appetite and cold hands and feet, plus symptoms of heart blood vacuity, such as a pale tongue, heart palpitations and insomnia. This formula is also the standard one for treating heavy or abnormal bleeding due to the spleen not containing and restraining the blood within its vessels. This patent medicine can be combined with *Xiao*

Yao Wan (see page 71) when there is liver depression qi stagnation complicated by heart blood and spleen qi vacuity. Its ingredients are:

Radix Astragali Membranacei *(Huang Qi)*
Radix Codonopsitis Pilosulae *(Dang Shen)*
Rhizoma Atractylodis Macrocephalae *(Bai Zhu)*
Sclerotium Parardicis Poriae Cocos *(Fu Shen)*
Mix-fried Radix Glycyrrhizae *(Gan Cao)*
Radix Angelicae Sinensis *(Dang Gui)*
Semen Zizyphi Spinosae *(Suan Zao Ren)*
Arillus Euphoriae Longanae *(Long Yan Rou)*
Radix Polygalae Tenuifoliae *(Yuan Zhi)*
Radix Auklandiae Lappae *(Mu Xiang)*

Er Chen Wan

Er Chen Wan means Two Aged (Ingredients) Pills. This is because two of its main ingredients are aged before using. This formula is used to transform phlegm and eliminate dampness. It can be added to *Xiao Yao Wan* (see page 71) if there is liver depression with spleen vacuity and more pronounced phlegm and dampness. Its ingredients include:

Rhizoma Pinelliae Ternatae *(Ban Xia)*
Sclerotium Poriae Cocos *(Fu Ling)*
Mix-fried Radix Glycyrrhizae *(Gan Cao)*
Pericarpium Citri Reticulatae *(Chen Pi)*
Uncooked Rhizoma Zingiberis *(Sheng Jiang)*

Ge Jie Da Bu Wan

This formula translates as Gecko Greatly Supplementing Pills and is designed to supplement the qi, blood, yin and yang. It is usually used to treat lower back and lower limb pain associated with kidney vacuity, in turn due to ageing. Since most women develop not only spleen vacuity but also kidney yin and yang vacuity as they move towards menopause in their late 40s, this formula can be combined with *Xiao Yao Wan* (see page 71) when there is liver depression, spleen and kidney yang vacuity and blood and yin vacuity as well. The ingredients in this Chinese patent medicine include:

Gecko *(Ge Jie)**
Radix Astragali Membranacei *(Huang Qi)*
Radix Codonopsitis Pilosulae *(Dang Shen)*
Fructus Lycii Chinensis *(Gou Qi Zi)*
Radix Angelicae Sinensis *(Dang Gui)*
Cooked Radix Rehmanniae *(Shu Di)*
Fructus Ligustri Lucidi *(Nu Zhen Zi)*
Rhizoma Polygonati *(Huang Jing)*
Rhizoma Atractylodis Macrocephalae *(Bai Zhu)*
Sclerotium Poriae Cocos *(Fu Ling)*
Radix Dioscoreae Oppositae *(Shan Yao)*
Radix Glycyrrhizae *(Gan Cao)*
Cortex Eucommiae Ulmoidis *(Du Zhong)*
Radix Dipsaci *(Xu Duan)*
Rhizoma Cibotii Barmetsis *(Gou Ji)**
Radix Morindae Officinalis *(Ba Ji Tian)*
Rhizoma Drynariae *(Gu Sui Bu)*
Fructus Chaenomelis Lagenariae *(Mu Gua)*

* *Ge Jie* is an animal product and *Gou Ji* is a listed endangered plant (trade is allowed with an appropriate permit). For those of you who wish to avoid these, a similar formula, Ganoderma 18, in the Seven Forest range, is available from the Number One Herb Co. (see page 155).

Jiang Ya Wan (also spelt *Chaing Ya Wan*)

Jiang Ya means to decrease pressure as in high blood pressure. *Wan*, as we have seen before, means pills. These pills are usually used to treat high blood pressure due to kidney vacuity and liver effulgence, but since Chinese medicine treats patterns of imbalance, rather than Western diseases as such, these pills can be used to treat PMS complaints such as headaches (including migraines), dizziness, red, painful eyes and irritability due to an upward flaring of liver fire or wind, in turn due to loss of control by kidney yin below. Since this formula already includes medicinals for treating the liver, it would not be combined with *Xiao Yao Wan* (see page 71) but used by itself. This formula contains several animal products; Cornu Antelopis Saiga-tatarici *(Ling Yang Jiao)* – antelope horn – and Gelatinum Corii Asini *(E Jiao)* – gelatine made from donkey hide. Its ingredients are:

Semen Leonuri Heterophyli *(Chong Wei Zi)*
Rhizoma Coptidis Chinensis *(Huang Lian)*
Cornu Antelopis Saiga-tatarici *(Ling Yang Jiao)**
Spica Prunellae Vulgaris *(Xia Ku Cao)*
Ramulus Uncariae Cum Uncis *(Gou Teng)*
Radix Gastrodiae Elatae *(Tian Ma)*
Succinum *(Hu Po)*
Radix Angelicae Sinensis *(Dang Gui)*
Radix Ligustici Wallichii *(Chuan Xiong)*
Uncooked Radix Rehmanniae *(Sheng Di)*
Gelatinum Corii Asini *(E Jiao)*
Cortex Radicis Moutan *(Dan Pi)*
Radix Achyranthis Bidentatae *(Niu Xi)*
Lignum Aquilariae Agallochae *(Chen Xiang)*
Radix Et Rhizoma Rhei *(Da Huang)*

* This ingredient is an endangered species listed by CITES and an appropriate trade permit is required.

Because this formula contains Radix Et Rhizoma Rhei (rhubarb), which is a strong purgative, it should not be taken if one has diarrhoea or loose stools. If this formula causes diarrhoea, its use should be discontinued.

ASSESSING OVER-THE-COUNTER MEDICATION

The previously mentioned patent formulae offer some suggestions as to how to treat your own PMS. Should you decide to do this, perhaps because there are no practitioners available in your area to give you guidance on Chinese herbs, then proceed with caution. Do not exceed the recommended dosage as given on the packet. If they do not work after three menstrual cycles or if you have any side-effects, then stop taking them immediately and try to get advice from a practitioner of Chinese herbal medicine. As mentioned previously, Chinese herbal medicines can be powerful and dynamic: they have the power to heal and therefore the potential to harm if incorrectly used. Follow the following guidelines for assessing the safety of any medications you take.

In general, you can tell if any medication and treatment is appropriate for you by checking the following six aspects of your health.

Digestion	Mood
Elimination	Appetite
Energy level	Sleep

If a medication, be it modern Western or traditional Chinese, alleviates your symptoms and these six areas of health also improve, then it is probably an appropriate treatment. However, if a treatment or medication causes a deterioration in any of these six mechanisms, even if there is an improvement in your symptoms, then it is probably not the correct treatment and certainly should not be taken on a long-term basis. Chinese medicine aims to rebalance the body's energies and create harmony, allowing the body's own natural healing mechanisms to be reinstated. Nothing is more powerful than nature's own healing and this is healing without side-effects.

ACUPUNCTURE AND ORIENTAL
MEDICAL MASSAGE

In the previous chapters we have looked at the underlying causes of PMS from a traditional Chinese medicine (TCM) point of view and its treatment with internal or herbal medicine. This chapter will focus on how Chinese medicine treats PMS using acupuncture and Oriental medical massage. Chinese medicine as it has evolved in China has developed in a different social and cultural context from the West and there are differences in how it is practised. In modern China, herbal treatment is very popular. In fact, TCM has evolved principally from a herbal tradition. In the West there have been many other influences and whilst TCM has played an important role, other countries have also been influential. Shiatsu, for example, a type of Oriental medical massage originating from Japan, is very popular in the West today and can be a very helpful therapy for PMS. Acupuncture is probably the most well known and widely practised form of Chinese medicine in the UK, having been practised since the 1960s. It has grown enormously in popularity and there are now many trained practitioners all over the UK. PMS in general responds very well to acupuncture, both on its own and combined with Chinese herbal medicine. We will look at how to find a properly qualified practitioner later on in the book.

ACUPUNCTURE

Acupuncture primarily means the insertion of extremely thin, sterilised, stainless steel needles into specific points on the body. These points are like switches for regulating and balancing the flow of qi and blood over the channel and network system we described earlier. As we have seen, PMS complaints are called menstrual movement diseases in Chinese medicine. This basically means that they are diseases caused by the incorrect flow of the qi and blood prior to the menses. As we have also seen, PMS and liver depression qi stagnation go hand in hand. The qi, which is depressed and stagnant, is not flowing when and where it should. Instead it counterflows or vents itself to inappropriate areas of the body, attacking other organs and body tissues and making them dysfunctional.

So, PMS typically includes many signs and symptoms associated with the lack or incorrect flow of qi. Since the real strength of acupuncture is its ability to regulate and rectify the flow of qi (and, by extension, the flow of blood since the qi moves the blood), it is particularly effective for treating menstrual movement diseases. The insertion of acupuncture needles at various points in the body moves the stagnant qi and leads the qi to flow in its proper directions and amounts.

As a generic term, acupuncture also includes several other methods of stimulating acupuncture points and regulating the flow of qi in the body. The other major modality is moxibustion, the stimulation of acupuncture points mainly by burning dried, aged Oriental mugwort on, near or over acupuncture points. The purposes of this warming treatment are to stimulate even more strongly the flow of qi and blood; to add warmth to areas of the body which are too cold; and to supplement the yang energy of the body. For full details see pages 126–28. Other methods of treatment used by acupuncturists are cupping (the application of suction cups over points), massage and bloodletting (pricking the points to allow a drop or two of blood to exit). Acupuncturists may also stimulate the points using medicinals or herbs, magnets and either electricity or laser.

Typical acupuncture treatments for PMS

In the USA and UK there are quite a few different styles of practising acupuncture so treatment will vary from one practitioner to another depending on their training. Practitioners may have trained according to Japanese, Vietnamese or Korean methods and this diversity of practice adds a great deal to the richness of acupuncture in the West. The style of practice that this book focuses on is traditional Chinese medicine (TCM) which is widely practised in the West and is the main method in modern China. It has evolved from a herbal tradition so the treatment principles are basically the same whether using herbs or acupuncture. It is by no means the only method of practising acupuncture so if your practitioner does not use this method it doesn't mean that it will be less effective. From the layperson's point of view, as long as you are seeing a properly qualified practitioner it doesn't really matter how they choose to practise as long as it works for you. Details are given on pages 145–48 about how to find a properly qualified practitioner.

Whatever kind of practitioner you choose, you will probably find that treatment is usually weekly or perhaps twice a week to start off with until the symptoms improve, and then less frequent. With PMS it will be necessary to work with your therapist for a few menstrual cycles but you will probably see some improvements quite quickly. Many people choose to continue having acupuncture to maintain their health once their original symptoms have cleared.

When you go to see your acupuncturist, the practitioner will ask you about all your symptoms and make a note of your medical history. They will feel the pulses at the radial arteries on both your wrists and may look at your tongue or examine your abdomen by gently palpating it. Based on their diagnosis, a number of acupuncture points are chosen for treatment.

The needles used nowadays are ethylene oxide gas-sterilised, disposable needles. This means that they are disposed of after each treatment session. Acupuncture needles are very fine, hardly thicker than a strand of hair and most are inserted only relatively shallowly into the skin. Make sure you see a properly qualified practitioner who follows sterile needle procedure, ensuring that there is absolutely no risk of infection from the needles.

After the needle has broken the skin, the acupuncturist will usually gently manipulate the needle to achieve the desired affect.

How are the points selected?

The points the acupuncturist chooses to stimulate in each treatment are selected on the basis of Chinese medical theory and the known clinical effects of certain points. Since there are different styles of acupuncture, the diagnosis and point selection will vary depending on your practitioner. Let me present a fairly typical case from a TCM point of view, as it is one of the most popular styles of practice.

Let's say for example that the woman's main complaints are premenstrual breast distension and pain (but no lumps or cystic tissue), irritability, fatigue and loose stools. Her tongue is swollen and pale, with thin, slightly slimy, white fur, and her pulse is fine and bowstring. Her Chinese pattern discrimination is premenstrual breast distension and pain, irritability and fatigue due to liver depression and spleen vacuity. This is a very commonly encountered scenario in women with PMS up to approximately 35 years of age.

The treatment principles necessary for remedying this case are to course the liver and rectify the qi, fortify the spleen and supplement the qi. Additionally, since breast distension and pain are major complaints, the practitioner will add treatment to loosen the chest and free the flow in the breasts.

In order to accomplish these aims, the practitioner might select the following points:

Tai Chong (Liver 3)
San Yin Jiao (Spleen 6)
Zu San Li (Stomach 36)
Ru Gen (Stomach 18)
Shan Zhong (Conception Vessel 17)
Pi Shu (Bladder 20)
Wei Shu (Bladder 21)

The rationale behind the choice of these points is as follows: *Tai Chong* courses the liver, resolves depression and moves and rectifies the qi. Since liver depression qi stagnation is the main disease mechanism causing this woman's PMS, this is the main or ruling point in this treatment. Since her irritability stems from liver depression, this point should really improve her symptoms.

San Yin Jiao is chosen to course the liver further and at the same time fortify the spleen. It does both these things because both the liver and spleen channels cross at this point. In addition, this point is known to be empirically effective for most urinogenital and reproductive problems. In Chinese medicine, it is said to possess a menstrual-regulating effect.

Zu San Li is one of the most powerful points on the stomach channel. As the stomach is the yang bowel relating to the yin spleen viscera, stimulating *Zu San Li* can bolster the spleen with yang qi from the stomach where it is usually plentiful. In addition, the stomach channel traverses the chest and, therefore, manipulation of needles at this point can regulate the qi in the chest and breasts in general.

Ru Gen is also on the stomach channel. It is located just under the breasts and is a local point for freeing and regulating the flow of qi through the breasts. *Shan Zhong*, which is located at the level of the nipples on the chest bone between the breasts, is another local point for freeing the flow of qi in the chest and breasts. This point is a special point for regulating the flow of qi in the entire body, but especially in the chest. It also helps calm the spirit and provide emotional relief.

Pi Shu and *Wei Shu* are both points on the back associated with the spleen and stomach respectively. They directly connect with this viscus and bowel and can supplement weakness and deficiencies in these two organs. In this case, the woman's fatigue and loose stools both stem from spleen vacuity and these two points have been proved to address both of these complaints.

This combination of seven points addresses the woman's Chinese pattern discrimination and her major complaints of breast distension and soreness, irritability, fatigue and loose stools. It both remedies the underlying disease mechanism and addresses certain key symptoms in a very direct and immediate way. Hence it provides symptomatic relief at the same time as correcting the underlying mechanisms of these symptoms.

Does acupuncture hurt?

In Chinese, it is said that acupuncture is *bu tong*, i.e. painless. Most patients will feel some sensation with the stimulation, but when done well and sensitively, it should not be sharp, biting, burning or really painful.

How quickly will I feel the result?

One of the best things about the acupuncture treatment of PMS is that its effects are immediate. Since many of the symptoms of PMS have to do with blocked qi, as soon as the qi is made to flow, the symptoms disappear. So, for many PMS complaints, such as breast distension and pain, headache, lower back pain, lower abdominal cramps, joint or muscle pain or epigastric pain, one may feel relief during the treatment itself.

In addition, because irritability and nervous tension are also mainly due to liver depression qi stagnation, most women will feel an immediate improvement in their general mood: irritability and tension may disappear whilst still lying on the treatment couch. Many people will feel a sense of pronounced tranquillity and relaxation within minutes.

Who should receive acupuncture?

Acupuncture is really beneficial to any woman experiencing PMS. It is particularly effective for breast distension and pain and in treating the mental and emotional tensions that are often very much part of PMS.

If the PMS symptoms are mostly a result of qi vacuity, blood vacuity, or yin vacuity, then acupuncture is not as effective as internally administered Chinese herbal medicinals. Although moxibustion (see page 126) can add yang qi to the body, acupuncture needles cannot add qi, blood or yin to someone who is depleted in these. The most that acupuncture can do in these cases is to stimulate the various viscera and bowels that engender and transform the qi, blood and yin. Chinese herbs, on the other hand, can directly introduce qi, blood and yin into the body, thus supplementing vacuities and deficiencies. In PMS cases, where qi, blood and yin vacuities are pronounced, you could use acupuncture either alone or combined with Chinese medicinals. When there is pronounced yang vacuity, you could use moxibustion alone or combine it with Chinese medicinals, but needles alone are unlikely to solve the problem.

Ear acupuncture

Some acupuncturists may also use points on the ear to treat PMS. Needles may be used during the acupuncture session or alternatively tiny metal pellets, seeds or special 'press tac' needles are used (these are then left in place for a few days after the treatment). In this way the effectiveness and duration of the treatment can be enhanced.

In terms of PMS, ear acupuncture is especially good for two things. First, stimulating the point known as *Shen Men* (Spirit Gate) can have a profound effect on relaxing tension and irritability and improving sleep. Secondly, needling the Mouth and/or Stomach points can to some degree decrease and control overeating and various cravings.

ORIENTAL MEDICAL MASSAGE

Medical massage in China is called *tui na*. It has developed into a high art and is practised extensively in hospitals and clinics. Like acupuncture, it works by stimulating the flow of qi in the channel or meridian system, except instead of needles, specific strokes or manipulations are used. At present, there are not many trained *tui na* practitioners in the UK, although it is growing in popularity. Another form of Oriental medical massage is Shiatsu, which originates from Japan. This is a deeply relaxing therapy and there are a number of practitioners working in the UK. Shiatsu is done with the patient wearing loose comfortable clothing. Diagnosis is mainly through palpating the abdomen and channels to detect underlying imbalances in the person's energy. The relevant channels or meridians are then worked on to release blockages and strengthen areas of vacuity or deficiency. It may be very beneficial for stress, which can affect PMS. Oriental medical massage can stimulate the flow of qi, and is particularly effective if you suffer from tension headaches as it is very relaxing.

THE THREE FREE THERAPIES

ll the treatments and therapies we have so far discussed require the aid of a professional practitioner. There are, however, three 'free' therapies that are crucial to preventing and treating PMS. These are diet, exercise and deep relaxation.

Remember that the root cause of PMS is likely to be liver depression qi stagnation. This is then typically complicated by spleen vacuity weakness. Liver depression arises primarily because of stress and emotional factors, while spleen vacuity is primarily due to poor diet. Of these three free therapies, therefore, diet is designed to support the spleen, and exercise and relaxation are meant to support the liver. If all three are co-ordinated and practised regularly, then they eliminate the causes and disease mechanisms of most cases of PMS. Diet in the West is, by Chinese medical standards, typically poor, and the Western way of life tends to be both excessively sedentary and excessively stressful, so the lack of proper management of these three basic realms of human life is the reason why PMS is so common. PMS has been around for millennia but its incidence is probably higher now in the West because of relatively recent changes in our diet and lifestyle.

DIET

In Chinese medicine, as I have said, the function of the spleen and stomach are likened to a pot on a stove or a still. The stomach receives the foods and liquids which then 'rot and ripen' like a mash in a fermentation vat. The spleen then cooks this mash and drives off (i.e. transforms and moves upwards) the pure part. This pure part collects in the lungs to become the qi and in the heart to become the blood. Chinese medicine characterises this transformation as a process of yang qi transforming yin substance. All the principles of Chinese dietary therapy that may be applied to treat and alleviate PMS are derived from these basic theories.

We have seen that a healthy spleen is vitally important for keeping the liver in check and the qi freely flowing. We have also seen that the spleen is the root of transformation and engenderment of qi and blood. Therefore, it is vitally important for women with PMS to avoid foods that damage the spleen and to eat foods that promote a healthy spleen and qi and blood production.

Foods that damage the spleen

The first of these are uncooked and especially chilled foods. In Chinese medicine the process of cooking is seen as a type of predigestion before the food enters the body. It is therefore desirable that the overwhelming majority of all food should be cooked, i.e. predigested. Although cooking may destroy some vital nutrients (in Chinese, qi), cooking does render the remaining nutrients more easily assimilated. This means that even though some nutrients have been lost, the net absorption of nutrients is greater with cooked foods than raw. Furthermore, eating raw foods makes the spleen work harder and can overtax it. If your spleen is very robust, eating uncooked, raw foods may not be too damaging; however, we have seen that many women's spleens are already weak because their monthly menses has overtaxed the spleen in regard to blood production.

Chilled foods may directly damage the spleen even more than raw foods. Chilled or frozen foods and drinks neutralise the spleen's yang qi. The process of digestion involves warming and digesting all food and drink to a warm soup within the stomach so that it may undergo 'distillation'. If the spleen expends too much yang qi just warming the food up, then it will become damaged and weak. So food and drink should be consumed at room temperature at the least and preferably at body temperature. The more signs and symptoms of spleen vacuity or deficiency a woman has – such as fatigue, chronically loose stools, undigested food in the stools, cold hands and feet, dizziness on standing up and aversion to cold – the more she needs to avoid uncooked, chilled foods and drinks.

Additionally, an excess of sugar and sweet things will directly damage the spleen. According to Chinese medicine, they are considered to be inherently dampening. This is because the body creates or secretes fluids that gather, transforming into dampness, in response to an excess of sweet food and drink. The spleen is averse to dampness. Dampness is a yin substance and controls or checks yang qi, which is very important to the proper functioning of the spleen. So anything that is excessively dampening damages the spleen. The sweeter a food is, the more dampening and therefore more damaging it is to the spleen.

Other food categories that are considered to be dampening and subsequently damaging to the spleen are:

'Sodden wheat' foods
This means flour products such as bread and noodles. Wheat (as opposed to rice) is damp in its nature. When it is steamed, yeasted and/or refined, it becomes even more damp.

Oils and fats
The more oily or greasy a food is, the worse it is for the spleen. As milk contains a lot of fat, dairy products fall into this category. This includes milk, butter and cheese.

If we add all this up, then ice cream is just about the worst thing a woman with a weak, damp spleen could eat. Ice cream is chilled, it is intensely sweet and it is filled with fat. So it is a triple whammy when it comes to damaging the spleen. Pasta smothered in tomato sauce and cheese is also a recipe for disaster. Pasta made from wheat flour is dampening, tomatoes are dampening and cheese is dampening. Fruit juice is also very damaging to the spleen and produces damp – most people don't realise that a glass of fruit juice contains as much sugar as a chocolate or sweet bar.

Below is a list of Western foods that are either uncooked, chilled, too sweet or too dampening and thus damaging to the spleen. Women with PMS should reduce their intake or avoid these, especially if they know their spleen is weak.

Ice cream
Sugar
Sweets, especially chocolate
Milk
Butter
Cheese
Margarine
Yoghurt
Raw salads
Fruit juices
Juicy, sweet fruits, such as oranges, peaches, strawberries and
    tomatoes
Fatty meats
Fried foods
Refined flour products
Cakes and biscuits
Yeasted bread
Nuts
Alcohol

If the spleen is weak and wet, it is best not to eat too much of anything at any one time. A weak spleen can be overwhelmed by a large meal, especially if any of the food is hard to digest.

This then results in food stagnation, which impedes the free flow of qi all the more and causes further damage to the spleen.

A clear, bland diet

In Chinese medicine, the best diet for the spleen and therefore, by extension, for most people, is what is called a 'clear, bland diet'. This is a diet high in complex carbohydrates such as unrefined grains, especially rice and beans. It is high in lightly cooked vegetables and low in fatty meats, oily, greasy, fried foods and very sweet foods. It is not, however, a completely vegetarian diet. Most women, in my experience, should eat 25–50 g / 1–2 oz of various types of meat two to four times per week. This animal flesh could be chicken and fish, but should also include some lean beef, pork and lamb. Some fresh or cooked fruits may be eaten, but fruit juices should be avoided. Women should make an effort to include tofu and tempeh in their diet, two soya foods now widely available in health food shops and major supermarkets.

If the spleen is weak, then it is best to eat smaller, more frequent meals. Rice is also an excellent food for three reasons: it is neutral in temperature, it fortifies the spleen thereby supplementing the qi, and it eliminates dampness. Rice should be the main grain in the diet.

A few problem foods

There are a few 'problem' foods that deserve special mention.

Coffee

Many people crave coffee for two reasons. Firstly, coffee moves blocked qi. So, if a person suffers from liver depression qi stagnation, coffee will temporarily make them feel as though their qi is flowing. Secondly, coffee transforms essence into qi and makes that qi temporarily available to the body.

This means that people who suffer from spleen and/or kidney vacuity fatigue will get a temporary lift from coffee. It will make them feel as though they have energy. However, once this energy is used up, they are left with a negative deficit. The coffee has transformed some of the essence stored in the kidneys into qi. This qi has been used and now there is less stored essence. Since the blood and essence share a common source, coffee drinking may ultimately worsen PMS associated with blood or kidney vacuities. Tea has a similar effect in that it transforms yin essence into yang qi, but the amount of caffeine in black tea is usually only half that found in coffee.

Chocolate

Chocolate is a combination of oil, sugar and cocoa. We have seen that both oil and sugar are dampening and damaging to the spleen. Sugar will boost the spleen qi temporarily, but ultimately it will result in 'sugar blues' or a hypoglycaemic let-down. Cocoa stirs the life gate fire, another name for kidney yang or kidney fire, and kidney fire is the source of sexual energy and desire. It is said that chocolate is the food of love and from the Chinese medical point of view, that is true. Since chocolate stimulates kidney fire at the same time as it temporarily boosts the spleen, it does give a rush of yang qi. This rush of yang qi does move stagnation, at least in the short term, so it makes sense that some women with liver depression, spleen vacuity and kidney yang debility might crave chocolate premenstrually.

Alcohol

Alcohol is both damp and hot according to Chinese medical theory. It strongly moves the qi and blood. So people with liver depression qi stagnation will feel temporarily better after drinking alcohol. The sugar in alcohol damages the spleen and creates dampness, which 'gums up the works', whilst the heat (yang) in alcohol can waste the blood (yin) and aggravate or inflame depressive liver heat.

Hot, peppery foods

Spicy, peppery, 'hot' foods also move the qi, thereby giving some temporary relief to liver depression qi stagnation. However, like alcohol, the heat in spicy, hot foods wastes the blood and can inflame yang.

Sour foods

In Chinese medicine, sour flavours are inherently astringent and constricting. People with liver depression qi stagnation should be careful not to use vinegar and other intensely sour foods, which will only aggravate the qi stagnation by further restricting the qi and blood. This is also why sweet and sour foods, such as orange juice and tomatoes, are particularly bad for women with liver depression spleen vacuity PMS. The sour flavour constricts the qi, while the sweet flavour damages the spleen and creates dampness.

Diet drinks

In my experience, diet drinks containing artificial sweeteners seem to contain something that damages the Chinese concept of the kidneys. A number of patients over the years have reported to me that when they drink a lot of diet drinks they experience urinary incontinence and soreness and weakness of the lower back and knees. If they stop, these symptoms disappear. Taken as a group, according to Chinese medicine, these are kidney vacuity symptoms. Since many women with PMS in their late 30s and through their 40s tend to have concomitant kidney vacuity, I recommend they steer clear of diet drinks so as not to weaken the kidneys any further or faster.

Diet, candidiasis and PMS

If you look at the diet I have recommended for women with PMS to eat, you will see that it is quite close to an anti-candida diet. Polysystemic chronic candidiasis (PSCC) refers to a chronic overgrowth of yeast and fungi in the body, which may affect many different systems in the body. The pathological changes associated with PSCC are due to a combination of food allergies, immune system imbalance and auto-immune reactions. In women, these pathological changes may affect the ovaries, adrenal glands, pituitary gland and thyroid gland. In Western women, a tendency towards PSCC is due to poor diet as outlined above, or overuse of antibiotics and hormone-based medicines, including oral birth control pills and corticosteroids. From a Chinese medical point of view, this then results in a deep-seated spleen vacuity with a damp encumbrance possibly complicated by liver depression, phlegm fluids, damp heat and/or blood stasis. If the spleen vacuity lasts long enough or is due to ageing, spleen vacuity may also involve kidney yang vacuity.

If a woman with PMS has a history of multiple fungal and yeast infections, together with recurrent or long-term antibiotic use (such as for recurrent bladder infections or pelvic inflammatory disease), and use of hormones as medicine, or if she suffers from allergies, PSCC should be suspected as a component of that woman's PMS. In that case, the woman should pay particular attention to her diet. The good news is that professionally prescribed Chinese herbal medicine can ease PSCC faster than just diet alone. The bad news is that, without proper diet, no amount of Chinese herbs will completely and permanently remedy this condition.

Vitamins

Vitamins and minerals can be very beneficial to women suffering from PMS, but they are not really relevant to a discussion of Chinese medicine. It is worth mentioning, however, that women with weak spleens should be careful about taking fatty acids for their PMS. As we have seen, oils are dampening and can easily damage the spleen. In my experience as a clinician, if you experience nausea or vomiting, indigestion or loose stools after taking such fatty acids, then these side-effects are because these oils have caused further dampening of the spleen. In this case, this supplement is not right for you. This is really one of the strengths of Chinese medicine and one of the major themes of this book. Chinese medicine allows the patient and their practitioner to determine if any treatment or food will be beneficial or harmful for them on the basis of their individual pattern discrimination.

Some last words on diet

In conclusion, Western patients are always asking me what they should eat in order to improve their condition. When it comes to diet, however, sad to say, the issue is not so much what to eat as what not to eat. Diet most definitely plays a major role in the cause and perpetuation of many women's PMS but, except in the case of vegetarians suffering from blood or yin vacuities, the issue is mainly what to avoid or reduce, not what to add. Most of us know that coffee, chocolate, sugars and sweets, oils, fats and alcohol are not good for us. Most of us know that we should be eating more complex carbohydrates and freshly cooked vegetables and less fatty meat. However, it's one thing to know these things and another to follow what we know by putting the theory into practice.

To be perfectly honest, a clear, bland diet as recommended according to the principles of Chinese medicine is not the most exciting diet in the world. However, it is quite a traditional diet, and many of our great-grandparents would have eaten like this. Our modern Western diet, which is high in oils and fats, high in sugars and sweets, high in animal proteins and proportionally high in uncooked, chilled foods and drinks, is a relatively recent phenomenon and you can't fool Mother Nature.

When you change to the clear, bland diet recommended by Chinese medicine, you might find that at first you suffer from cravings for more tasty food. These cravings are, in many cases, actually associated with food 'allergies'. We crave foods that are actually not good for us in the same way that an alcoholic craves alcohol. After a few days, these cravings tend to disappear and you can find that you don't miss some of the convenience or 'comfort' foods as much as you thought you would. Perseverance is the key to long-term success. As the Chinese say, 'A million is made up of nothing but lots of ones and a bucket is quickly filled by steady drops.'

EXERCISE

Exercise is the second of the three free therapies. According to Chinese medicine, regular and adequate exercise has two basic benefits. Firstly, exercise promotes the movement of the qi and quickening of the blood. Since all PMS involves at least some component of liver depression qi stagnation, it is obvious that exercise is an important therapy for coursing the liver and rectifying the qi. Secondly, exercise benefits the spleen. The spleen's movement and transportation of digested food is dependent upon the qi mechanism. The qi mechanism describes the function of the qi in moving up and down the pure and turbid parts of digestion respectively. For the qi mechanism to function properly, the qi must be flowing normally and freely. Since exercise moves and rectifies the qi, it also helps regulate and rectify the qi mechanism. The result is that the spleen is able to function well, creating and transforming qi and blood. Spleen vacuity and qi and blood vacuity typically complicate most women's PMS, and because a healthy spleen controls and keeps in check a depressed liver, exercise treats the other most commonly encountered disease mechanism in the majority of cases of PMS. Regular and adequate exercise is a vitally important component of any woman's regime for either preventing or treating PMS.

Aerobics

In my experience, aerobic exercise is found to be most beneficial for the majority of women with PMS. By aerobic exercise, I mean any physical activity that raises your heartbeat 80 per cent above your normal resting rate and keeps it there for at least 20 minutes. To calculate your normal resting heart rate, place your fingers over the pulsing artery on the front side of your neck. Count the beats for 15 seconds and then multiply by four. This gives you your beats per minute, or BPM. Now multiply your BPM by 0.8. Take the resulting number and add it to your resting BPM. This gives you your aerobic threshold of BPM. Next engage in any physical activity you like. After you have been exercising for five minutes, take your pulse for 15 seconds once again at the artery on the front side of your throat. Again multiply the resulting count by four and this tells you your current BPM. If this number is less than your aerobic threshold BPM, then you know you need to exercise harder or faster. Once you get your heart rate up to your aerobic threshold, then you need to keep exercising at the same level of intensity for at least 20 minutes. Take your pulse every five minutes or so to ensure your heart rate is being kept high enough.

Depending on your age and physical condition, you will require different amounts and types of aerobic exercise to reach your aerobic threshold. For some people, simply walking briskly will raise their heart rate 80 per cent above its resting rate. Others will need to do calisthenics, running, swimming, squash or some other more strenuous exercise. It really does not matter what the exercise is as long as it raises your heartbeat 80 per cent above your resting rate and keeps it there for 20 minutes. The essential thing is that you go for something you enjoy, otherwise you will have a hard time keeping it up. You should also try to make sure that it doesn't cause any damage to any parts of the body. For example, running on pavements may cause knee problems for some people.

When doing aerobic exercise, it is best to exercise either every day or every other day. Unless aerobics are done at least once every 72 hours, the cumulative effects will not be as great. I recommend that my patients with PMS do some sort of aerobic exercises three to four times per week at least. The good news is that there is no real need to exercise for more than 30 minutes at any one time. A session of 45 minutes is not going to be all that much better than one of 25 minutes. And 25 minutes four times per week is much better than one hour once a week.

Recent research has also demonstrated that weight-lifting can help relieve depressive symptoms of PMS in women of all ages. It might be beneficial to try and schedule some weight-lifting into your exercise routine. I suggest that you do aerobics three to four days a week and lift weights on the other three days. In general, it is not a good idea to lift weights every day unless you vary the muscle groups you are working with each day. In a study on weight-lifting and depression, the women lifted weights that were 45–87 per cent of the maximum weight they could lift at one time. Those women who lifted weights closer to the top end of this range saw the greatest benefits. These women lifted weights three days per week for 10 weeks, gradually increasing the amount of weight they lifted at each session.

Weight-lifting requires training in order to do it safely and properly, so you will need to take a few classes at a local gym, sports club or recreation centre or from a personal trainer. When aerobic and weight-lifting sessions are alternated, you have a really comprehensive training regime designed to benefit the cardiovascular system, muscles, tendons, ligaments and bones. Regular weight-bearing exercise is also important for preventing osteoporosis.

DEEP RELAXATION

As we have seen, PMS is associated with liver depression qi stagnation. Typically, the worse the PMS is, the worse the woman's liver depression. This condition arises because of emotional upset, frustration and stress, which is why a certain amount of liver depression is endemic amongst all adults. When qi becomes depressed in the liver, it accumulates like hot air in a balloon. Eventually, this hot, depressed, angry qi has to go somewhere. So if there is further frustration or stress, then this angry qi in the liver explodes as irritability, anger or shouting.

Essentially, this type of anger and irritability is due to a maladaptive coping response that is typically learned at a young age. When we feel frustrated or stressed about something, most of us tense our muscles, and especially the muscles in our upper back and shoulders, neck and jaws. At the same time, many of us will hold our breath. In Chinese medicine, the sinews are governed by the liver. This tensing of the sinews, i.e. the muscles, constricts the flow of qi in the channels and network vessels. Since it is the liver that is responsible for the coursing and discharging of this qi, such tensing of the sinews leads to liver depression qi stagnation. Because the lungs govern the downward spreading and movement of the qi, holding our breath due to stress or frustration only worsens this tendency of the qi not to move and, therefore, to become depressed in the Chinese medical idea of the liver.

This is why deep relaxation is the third of the three free therapies. For deep relaxation to be therapeutic medically, it needs to be more than just mental equilibrium. It needs to be somatic (bodily) relaxation as well as mental repose. Most of us don't realise that every thought we think and feeling we feel is actually felt as a physical sensation somewhere in our body. The words we use to describe emotions are all abstract nouns, such as anger, depression, sadness and melancholy. However, in Chinese medicine, every emotion is associated with a change in the direction or flow of qi. For instance, anger makes the qi move upwards, while fear makes it move downwards. Therefore, anger 'makes our gorge rise' or makes us 'blow our top', while fear may cause a 'sinking feeling'. These colloquial expressions are all based on the age-old wisdom that all thoughts and emotions are not just mental but also physical events. This is why it is not just enough to clear one's mind. Clearing the mind is good, but for really marked therapeutic results it is even better to clear the mind at the same time as relaxing one's breathing and every muscle in the body.

Guided, deep relaxation tapes

An effective way to practise such mental and physical deep relaxation is to listen to a daily, guided, progressive, deep relaxation audiotape. It is guided in the sense that a narrator on the tape leads you through the process of deep relaxation. These tapes normally lead you to relax the body in a progressive manner, first relaxing one part and then moving on to another.

There are many such tapes available, usually sold in health food shops or good bookshops. Choose several tapes so that you won't get too bored of listening to the same one. When looking for a good relaxation tape, firstly ensure that the tape is a guided tape and not a subliminal relaxation tape. Subliminal tapes usually have music, and any instructions to relax are given so quietly that they are not consciously heard. Although such tapes can help you feel relaxed when you listen to them, ultimately they do not teach you relaxation as a skill that you can then consciously practise.

Secondly, make sure the tape starts from the top of the body and works downwards. This is because anger makes the qi go upwards in the body, even when frustration and anger due to liver depression qi stagnation means there is already too much qi rising upwards in the body. This depressed qi needs not only to be moved but to be moved downwards.

Thirdly, make sure the tape instructs you to relax your physical body. If you do not relax all your muscles, the qi cannot flow freely and the liver cannot be coursed. The tape will not be as beneficial if you don't relax your muscles.

Finally, try to make sure the tape instructs you to breathe out with each exhalation. One of the symptoms of liver depression is a stuffy feeling in the chest that we then unconsciously try to relieve by sighing. Letting each exhalation go completely helps the lungs push the qi downwards.

The importance of daily practice

I was once taken on a field trip to a Shanghai clinic where they were using deep relaxation as a therapy with patients with high blood pressure, heart disease, stroke, migraines and insomnia. The doctors at this clinic produced various graphs plotting their research data on how such daily, progressive, deep relaxation can regulate the blood pressure and body temperature and improve the appetite, digestion, elimination, sleep, energy and mood. One of the things they said has stuck with me since then: 'Small results in 100 days, big results in 1,000.' This means that if one does such daily, progressive deep relaxation every single day for 100 days, one will definitely experience results. These 'small' results are improvements in blood pressure, body temperature, appetite, digestion, elimination, sleep, energy and mood. The 'big' results experienced in 1,000 days of practice are more fundamental and permanent; they really are about a change in how one reacts to stress, and are much more permanent.

What these doctors in Shanghai stressed – and I have experienced this both personally and with my patients – is that the effects of this relaxation are cumulative, meaning that the longer one can practise this routine on a consistent daily basis, the greater and more lasting the effects will be.

It is vitally important to do such daily, guided, progressive, deep relaxation on a daily basis for at least three months and ideally for three years. If you achieved this goal, then you would see improvement in every parameter of your health and well-being. If you do this kind of deep relaxation sporadically, missing a day here and there, it will have some benefit, but it will not have the marked, cumulative therapeutic effects that are possible.

The real test

Doing a daily deep relaxation regime is only practice, however. It's like hitting tennis balls against a wall or hitting a bucket of balls at a driving range; it's not the real thing. The real purpose of a daily deep relaxation regime is not just to relieve the immediate stress and strain but to learn a new skill, a new way to react to stress. The ultimate goal is to recondition the way you react in stressful situations, and involves learning how to breathe out and relax your muscles rather than holding your breath and tensing your muscles. This is the real test, the game of life. Remember: 'Small results in 100 days, big results in 1,000.'

FINDING THE TIME

If you're like me and most of my patients, you are probably saying to yourself right now, 'This is all well and good, but when am I supposed to find the time to eat well-balanced cooked meals, exercise at least every other day and do a deep relaxation every day? I'm already stretched to the limit.'

As a clinician, I often wish I could wave a magic wand over my patients' heads and make them all healthy and well. I cannot. After almost 20 years of working with thousands of patients, I know of no easy way to health. There is good living and there is easy living and the so-called line of least resistance is actually going to make the situation worse. Unless you take time for yourself and find the time to eat well, exercise and relax, no treatment is going to eliminate your PMS completely. There is simply no pill you can pop or food you can eat that will get rid of the root causes of PMS: poor diet, too little exercise and too much stress. Even Chinese herbal medicine and acupuncture will only have their full effect if the diet and lifestyle are adjusted first. Sun Si-maio, the most famous Chinese doctor of the Tang dynasty (618–907 AD), who lived to be 101, said: 'First adjust the diet and lifestyle and only secondarily give herbs and acupuncture.' Similarly, Chinese medicine nowadays recommends: 'Three parts treatment, seven parts nursing.' For 'nursing', read 'proper diet and lifestyle'.

In my experience, this is absolutely true. The majority of all conditions will improve after three months of proper diet, exercise, relaxation and lifestyle modification. Each of us has certain rituals we perform each day, for instance, brushing our teeth, having a shower or eating a good lunch. And 99.99 per cent of us find or make the time to get dressed each day. The same applies to good eating, exercise and deep relaxation. Where there's a will, there's a way. If your PMS is bad enough, you can make the time to eat well, take proper exercise and enjoy a daily session of deep relaxation.

THE SOLUTION TO PMS IS IN YOUR HANDS

Where I live, we have a pedestrian centre in town. On summer evenings, my wife and I often walk down this mall. Having treated so many patients over the years, it is not unusual for me to meet former patients on these strolls. Frequently when we say hello, these patients begin by telling me they are sorry they haven't been in to see me for such a long time. They usually say this apologetically, as if they have done something wrong. I then usually ask if they've been all right. Often they tell me: 'When my problem flares up, I remember what you told me about my diet, exercise and lifestyle. I then go back to doing my exercise or deep relaxation or I change my diet and my symptoms just go away. That's why I haven't been in. I'm sorry.'

These patients have no need to apologise. This kind of story is music to my ears. When I hear that these patients are now able to control their own conditions by following the dietary and lifestyle advice I gave them, I know that, as a doctor of Chinese medicine, I have done my job correctly. According to Chinese medicine, a doctor who treats disease after it has appeared is not a good doctor. A good doctor prevents disease before it has arisen. If I can teach my patients how to cure their symptoms by making changes in their diet and lifestyle, then I'm approaching the goal of the best Chinese doctor – the prevention of disease through patient education.

The professional practice of medicine is a strange business. We doctors are, or at least should be, always engaged in putting ourselves out of business. Therefore, patients have no need to apologise to me when they tell me they now have control over their health.

So, to feel real benefit, you need to make the necessary changes in eating and behaviour. In addition, PMS is not a condition that is cured once and for all, like measles or mumps. When I say Chinese medicine can cure PMS, I do not mean that you will never experience premenstrual symptoms again. What I mean is that Chinese medicine can eliminate or greatly reduce your symptoms as long as you keep your diet and lifestyle together. People being people, we all 'fall off the wagon' from time to time and we all 'choose our own poisons'. I do not expect perfection from either my patients or myself. Therefore, I am not looking for a lifetime cure. Rather, I try to give my patients an understanding of what causes their conditions and what they can do to minimise or eliminate their causes and mechanisms. It is then up to the patient to decide what is bearable and what is unbearable, or what is an acceptable level of health. The Chinese doctors will have done their job when you know how to correct your health and are prepared to accept the price you have to pay.

SIMPLE HOME REMEDIES FOR PMS

lthough, according to Chinese medicine, poor diet, lack of adequate exercise and too much stress are the ultimate causes of PMS, and therefore diet, exercise and deep relaxation are the most important parts of every woman's treatment and prevention of PMS, there are also simple Chinese home remedies that will to help relieve the symptoms.

CHINESE AROMATHERAPY

In Chinese medicine, the qi is seen as a type of wind or vapour. The Chinese character for qi shows wind blowing over a rice field. In addition, the smell of something is often referred to as its qi. Therefore, there is a close relationship between smells carried through the air and the flow of qi in a person's body. Although aromatherapy has not been a major part of professionally practised Chinese medicine for almost 1,000 years, there is a simple aromatherapy treatment that you can do at home to help alleviate premenstrual irritability, depression, nervousness, anxiety and insomnia.

In Chinese, *Chen Xiang* means 'sinking fragrance'. It is the name of Lignum Aquilariae Agallochae (eaglewood). This is a frequent ingredient in Asian incense formulae. In Chinese medicine, Aquilaria is classified as a qi-rectifying medicinal. When used as a boiled decoction or tea, Aquilaria moves the qi and stops pain, moves down upward counterflow and regulates the middle (i.e. the spleen and stomach), and promotes the kidneys' grasping of the qi sent down by the lungs. I believe that the word 'sinking' in this herb's name refers to this medicinal's moving down upwardly counterflowing qi. Such qi must eventually accumulate in the heart, disturbing and causing restlessness of the heart spirit. When this medicinal wood is burnt and its smoke is inhaled as a medicinal incense, its bearing-down and spirit-calming function is emphasised.

You can buy Aquilaria *(Chen Xiang)* from specialist Chinese herbal suppliers or shops. It is best to use the powdered variety. However, you can grind it yourself in a coffee grinder or you can use small pieces of the herb if powder is not available. You will also need a roll of incense charcoals. Place one charcoal in a flameproof dish and light it with a match. Then sprinkle a few pinches of Aquilaria powder on the lit charcoal. As the smoke rises, breathe in deeply. This can be done on a regular basis several times per day during the premenstruum or as required by those suffering from restlessness, nervousness, anxiety, irritability and depression. For those who experience premenstrual insomnia, you can carry out this treatment when lying in bed at night.

Chinese aromatherapy with Lignum Aquilariae Agallochae is very effective and I have not heard of any side-effects or contraindications.

MAGNET THERAPY

The Chinese have used magnet therapy since at least the Tang dynasty (618–907 AD). Placing magnets on the body is a painless way of stimulating acupuncture points without inserting needles through the skin. Since magnets can be taped on to points and worn for days at a time, Chinese magnet therapy is able to provide easy, low-cost, continuous treatment. Below are magnetic treatments for menstrual irregularities, including early, delayed and erratic menstruation, excessive and scanty menstruation, lower abdominal pain occurring either before or at the onset of the period, and premenstrual breast distension and pain.

Suppliers of special adhesive magnets for stimulating acupuncture points, such as Acu-Band Magnets, Corimag or Epaule Patch TDK Magnets, are given on pages 152–56. The magnets range in strength from 400 to 9,000 gauss, the unit measuring magnetic strength. For the treatments below, you could try 400–800 gauss magnets.

Magnet therapy for menstrual irregularities

Tape small body magnets over the following points. Place the south pole in contact with the skin if the condition is due to liver depression qi stagnation, depressive liver heat or blood stasis. Place the north pole against the skin if the condition is due to spleen, liver or kidney vacuities. Leave the magnets in place for three to five days at a time, then remove for one day so that the body does not become habituated to this stimulation. Reapply for another three to five days as needed.

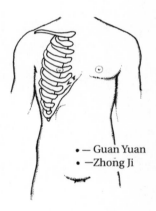

Guan Yuan (Conception Vessel 4): This point is located on the midline of the lower abdomen four finger-breadths below the navel. It connects directly to both the kidneys and the uterus.

Zhong Ji (Conception Vessel 3): This point is located on the midline of the lower abdomen five finger-breadths below the navel. It also connects with the uterus.

• — Guan Yuan
• —Zhong Ji

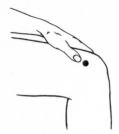

Xue Hai (Spleen 10): This point is located approximately 5 cm/2 in above the upper, inside edge of the kneecap when the knee is bent. This point's name means Sea of Blood and so it is used to treat all blood diseases, especially heat in the blood and static blood.

San Yin Jiao (Spleen 6): This point is located 7.5 cm/3 in above the tip of the inner ankle bone on the back edge of the tibia or shin bone. It is an intersection point of the spleen, liver and kidney channels, which all 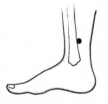 enter the uterus. It is used to treat all urinogenital and reproductive tract disorders. It has a very broad regulating action on menstruation.

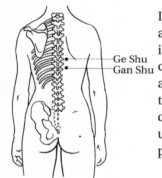

In case of breast distension and pain, add *Gan Shu* (Bladder 18). This point is located 4 cm/1½ in lateral to the centre of the spine at the same level as the lower edge of the ninth thoracic vertebra. This point connects directly with the liver and is used to treat diseases due to liver patterns of disharmony.

In case of early menstruation with purplish blood clots due to depressive heat and blood stasis, add *Ge Shu* (Bladder 17). This point is located 4 cm/1½ in lateral to the centre of the spine at the same level as the lower edge of the seventh thoracic vertebra.

Magnet therapy for lower abdominal pain associated with menstruation

Tape small body magnets over the following points. In case of repletion patterns of liver depression, damp heat, depressive heat and blood stasis, the south pole should touch the skin. In case of vacuity patterns of the spleen, liver and/or kidneys, the north pole should touch the skin. Apply three days before the expected onset of the period and leave in place until after the time the menstrual pain would ordinarily have ceased.

Guan Yuan (Conception Vessel 4): see page 111.
Zhong Ji (Conception Vessel 3): see page 111.

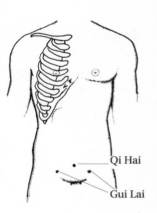

Qi Hai (Conception Vessel 6): This point is located two finger-breadths below the navel on the midline of the lower abdomen. Its name means Sea of Qi and it governs the qi of the entire body and especially of the lower abdomen.

Gui Lai (Stomach 29): This point is located 5 cm/2 in to either side of *Zhong Ji* (see page 111). It is primarily used for qi stagnation and blood stasis pain associated with menstruation.

Qi Hai

Gui Lai

San Yin Jiao (Spleen 6): see page 112.

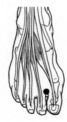

In case of qi stagnation, add *Xing Jian* (Liver 2). This point is located just above the web between the large and second toes on the top of the foot. It is the drainage point of the liver and thus drains liver depression qi stagnation and depressive liver heat.

In case of vacuity cold, add *Ming Men* (Governing Vessel 4). This point is located in the centre of the spine just below the lower edge of the second lumbar vertebra. *Ming Men* means Life Gate and refers to the life gate fire or kidney yang. Thus this point supplements the kidneys and invigorates yang. The north side of the magnet should generally touch the skin at this point. In case of early menstruation with purplish blood clots due to blood heat and stasis, add *Ge Shu* (Bladder 17). See page 112.

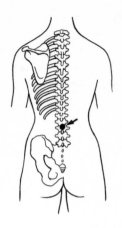

Magnet therapy for premenstrual breast distension and pain, and fibrocystic breasts

Tape small body magnets over the following points. Since most breast disease is at least locally a repletion or excess condition, tape the south poles in contact with the skin. Leave in place for three to five days, then remove and take a rest for one day to prevent the body from habituating to the stimulation. Reapply as needed.

Jian Jing (Gall Bladder 21): This point is located at the high point in the top centre of the trapezius or shoulder muscle. It effectively reverses upwardly counterflowing qi.

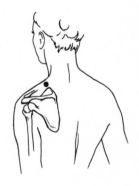

Hou Xi (Small Intestine 3): This point is located on the side of the hand below the little finger where the heart line meets the back of the hand. This point is known to have a very strong empirical effect on breast diseases due to counterflowing qi caused by depression.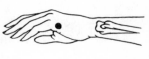

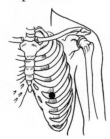 *Ru Gen* (Stomach 18): This point is located directly beneath the nipple in the fifth intercostal space. It frees the flow of qi locally in the breasts and is used for a variety of breast diseases.

Zu San Li (Stomach 36): This point is located 7.5 cm/3 in below the lower outside edge of the kneecap. It regulates the qi of the entire body and especially of the stomach channel which traverses the breasts.

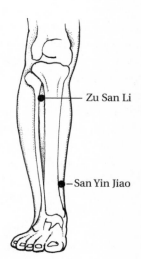

San Yin Jiao (Spleen 6): This point is located 7.5 cm/3 in above the inner ankle bone. See also page 112.

If there are any cystic lumps, also tape a magnet with the south pole touching the skin directly over these.

Should your symptoms worsen whilst using magnets, remove them and seek professional guidance from an acupuncturist.

LIGHT THERAPY

Light therapy, more specifically sunbathing or heliotherapy, is one of Chinese medicine's health preservation and longevity practices. Sunlight is considered the most essential yang qi in nature. Li Shi-zhen, one of the most famous Chinese doctors of the late Ming dynasty (1368–1644 AD), wrote, '*Tai yang* (literally, 'supreme yang' but also a name for the sun) is true fire.' As he pointed out, 'Without fire, heaven is not able to engender things and without fire, people are not able to live.' Since the back of the human body is yang (as compared to the front which is more yin), exposing the back to sunlight is a good way of increasing the yang qi of the body.

As we have seen, most women's yang qi begins to decline by around 35 years of age. In women over 35, most premenstrual fatigue, loose stools, lack of strength, poor memory, lack of concentration, poor co-ordination, decline in or lack of libido, lower back and knee soreness and weakness, increased night-time urination and cold hands and feet are due to an initial decline in the yang qi of the spleen and later in the yang qi of the spleen and kidneys. When many women say they are depressed, they can often mean in Chinese medical terms that they are extremely fatigued. In these sorts of cases, sunbathing can help supplement the yang qi of the body, thereby strengthening the spleen and/or kidneys.

Furthermore, because the yang qi is also the motivating force that pushes the qi, increasing yang qi can also help resolve depression and move stagnation. Cao Ting-dong, a famous doctor of the Qing dynasty (1644–1911 AD), wrote: 'Sitting with the back exposed directly to the sun, the back may get warmed. This is able to make the entire body harmonious and smoothly flowing. The sun is the essence of *tai yang* and its light strengthens the yang qi of the human body.'

In Chinese medicine, the words harmonious and smoothly flowing together refer to the flow of qi and blood. Hence, sunbathing can help course the liver and rectify the qi as well as fortify the spleen and invigorate the kidneys.

It has been said that sunlight is good for every disease except skin cancer. As we now know, overexposure to the sun can cause skin cancer through sunlight damaging the cells of the skin. Therefore, you should be careful not to get too much sun and not to get sunburnt. According to Chinese medicine, sunbathing should be done between the hours of 8 a.m. and 10 a.m. Sunbathing between 11 a.m. and 1 p.m. in winter is recommended only in temperate, not tropical, latitudes.

It is interesting to note, however, that some Western researchers are beginning to understand that exposure to light does play a role in relieving many women's PMS.

HYDROTHERAPY

Hydrotherapy means water therapy and is a part of traditional Chinese medicine. There are numerous different water treatments for helping to relieve various symptoms of PMS, one of the simplest being a warm bath. If you take a warm bath just slightly higher than body temperature for 15–20 minutes, this can free and smooth the flow of qi and blood. In addition, it can relieve premenstrual tension and irritability, calm the spirit and hasten sleep. Taking a warm bath half an hour before going to bed can help premenstrual insomnia.

However, when taking a warm bath, you must be careful not to use water so hot or to stay in the bath so long that sweat breaks out on your forehead. We lose yang qi as well as body fluids when we sweat. As fluids and blood share a common source, excessive sweating can cause problems for women with blood and yin vacuities. Sweating can also worsen yang qi vacuities in women whose spleen and kidneys are weak.

Therefore, unless they are given a specific hot bath prescription by their Chinese medical practitioner, I suggest women with PMS should not stay in warm baths until they sweat. Although they may feel pleasantly relaxed, they may later feel excessively fatigued or hot and thirsty. The latter is especially the case in women who are menopausal. In these women, hot baths may increase hot flushes and night sweats.

If, due to depression transforming heat, yang qi is exuberant and counterflowing upwards, it may cause premenstrual migraines and tension headaches, hot flushes, night sweats, painful, red eyes or even nosebleeds. In these cases, you can soak your feet in cold water for 15–20 minutes at a time. You may also soak your hands in cold water, or put a cold, wet compress on the back of your neck. The first two treatments seek to draw yang qi away from the head either to the lower part of the body or out to the extremities. The third treatment seeks to block and neutralise yang qi from counterflowing upwards, congesting in the head and damaging the blood vessels in the head.

For women who either catch cold before each period or are struggling with obesity, one can use cool baths, slightly lower than body temperature, for 10 minutes per day. Although this may seem contradictory, since cold is yin and these patients already suffer from a yang insufficiency, this brief and not too extreme exposure to cool water stimulates the body to produce more yang qi. In the case of premenstrual colds and flu, I would only do this treatment after ovulation and up to the onset of the menses. In the case of obesity due to a low metabolic rate, one can take cool baths from the cessation of menstruation to its onset. According to Chinese medicine, it is not advisable to take cold baths during menstruation itself as this may retard the free flow of qi and blood and lead to dysmenorrhoea or painful menstruation.

For painful menstruation due to qi stagnation and blood stasis, you can apply warm, wet compresses to the lower abdomen for 15–20 minutes at a time. You should not sleep with a hot water bottle or heating pad. If you use such a hot application for too long, it begins to raise the body temperature. The body must maintain its normal temperature of 37°C/98.6°F. Therefore, if the body temperature rises due to local application of heat, the body's response is actually to cut off the blood flow to that area of the body. This would then result in just the opposite effect from the one we want.

Warm, wet compresses can be applied to the breasts for the relief of premenstrual breast distension and pain. In either case, simmering several slices of fresh ginger in the water for five to seven minutes and then using the resulting infusion to make the hot compress can increase the effect of moving the qi and quickening the blood.

CHINESE SELF-MASSAGE

Massage, including self-massage, is a highly developed part of traditional Chinese medicine. At its most basic, rubbing promotes the flow of qi and blood in the area rubbed. On the next few pages are three Chinese self-massage regimes. The first is for headache, the second for menstrual irregularities in general and the third for premenstrual breast distension and pain. In fact, there are Chinese self-massage regimes for diarrhoea, constipation, nausea and vomiting, acne, all sorts of body pain, colds and flu, insomnia, dizziness and painful menstruation. All of these may be used premenstrually by women with PMS.

Self-massage for headache

1. Begin by pressing and kneading the area between the eyebrows above the bridge of the nose. This is the acupuncture point *Yin Tang* and is especially useful for calming the spirit and soothing the liver. Do this approximately 100 times.

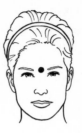

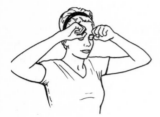

2. Rub the eyebrows with the thumbs and forefingers from the centre outward. Do this 100 times.

3. Rub the temples with the tips of the thumbs or middle fingers 100 times until there is a feeling of mild soreness and distension.

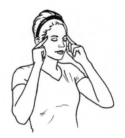

4. Rub the temples backward with the edges of the thumbs, from the orbits of the eyes to within the hairline 100 times. Rub in only one direction, from front to back.

5. Place the fingers of one hand on the forehead so that the middle finger is in the middle of the forehead and the other fingers are just below the hairline to either side. The palm of the hand will be resting gently on the top of the head. Now massage backwards from the forehead to the centre of the top of the head 20–30 times. The hands should move backwards by tightening and relaxing the fingertips.

6. Pat the top of the head with the hollow of the palm 30–50 times. The point in the middle of the top of the head is called *Bai Hui* (Meeting of Hundreds, Governing Vessel 20). Stimulation of this point calms the spirit and reverses upwardly counterflowing and exuberant liver yang.

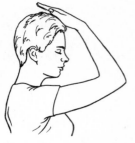

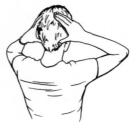

7. Press and knead the base of the skull in the depressions on both sides of the back of the neck. This is acupuncture point *Feng Chi* (Gall Bladder 20) and is a major point for relieving headache due to upwardly counterflowing liver qi. Do this approximately 100 times.

8. Lightly pound the centre of the top of one shoulder with the fist of the opposite hand. This is acupuncture point *Jian Jing* (Gall Bladder 21). It also downbears upwardly counterflowing liver qi. Do this 30–50 times on each side.

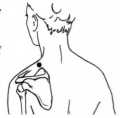

This self-massage regime is appropriate for premenstrual migraines and other types of headaches due to the upward counterflow of liver yang, depressive heat or liver wind and/or fire.

Self-massage for menstrual irregularities

Menstrual irregularities include early menstruation, delayed menstruation, erratic menstruation, excessive menstruation and scanty menstruation. The term can also be used for premenstrual spotting and premenstrual lower abdominal bloating and pain.

1. Begin by pressing and kneading each of three points 100 times. First press and knead *Zhong Wan* (Conception Vessel 12). This point is located on the midline of the abdomen, halfway between the lower tip of the sternum and the navel. Next press and knead *Qi Hai* (Conception Vessel 6). This point is on the midline of the lower abdomen, two finger-breadths below the navel. Then press and knead *Guan Yuan* (Conception Vessel 4). This point is located four finger-breadths below the navel on the midline of the lower

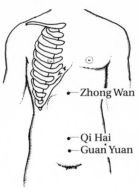

abdomen. *Zhong Wan* regulates the spleen and stomach, the root of qi and blood engenderment and transformation. *Qi Hai* regulates the qi in the entire body and especially in the uterus. *Guan Yuan* also connects directly to the uterus and regulates menstruation.

2. Press and knead all down the large muscles on either side of the spine. Press and knead approximately 4 cm/1½ in on either side of the spine. There are acupuncture points along the spine that connect directly with all the viscera and bowels. The production and function of the qi and blood is dependent on the proper functioning of the viscera and bowels, and regular menstruation depends on the proper production and function of the qi and blood.

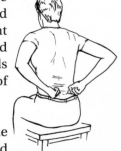

3. Press and knead the sacrum. Points on the sacrum connect directly with the uterus and so regulate menstruation.

4. Press and knead three points 50–100 times each on the lower legs. The first point is *Zu San Li* (Stomach 36). This point is located 7.5 cm/3½ in below the lower, outside edge of the kneecap. This point regulates the qi of the entire body, regulates the qi of the stomach channel in particular and fortifies the spleen at the same time as it harmonises the stomach. The second point is *Xue Hai* (Spleen 10). Its name means Sea of Blood. Therefore, this point has a regulatory effect on the blood of the entire body. Since menstruation is a flow and discharge of blood, stimulating this point helps to quicken the blood and

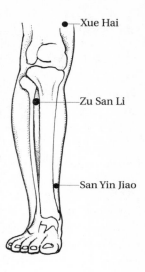

dispel stasis. It is located approximately 5 cm/2 in above the upper, inside edge of the kneecap when the knee is bent. The third point is *San Yin Jiao* (Spleen 6). This point is an intersection of the spleen, liver and kidney channels, all three of which connect directly with the uterus. It is used for all urinogenital and reproductive tract diseases. It is located 7.5 cm/3 in above the tip of the inner ankle bone on the back edge of the tibia or shin bone.

5. Rub and pat the lower back or lumbar region. First rub the lumbar region back and forth from side to side until the area becomes warm to the touch. Then pat the area with the hollow of both palms 30–50 times. The lower back is called the mansion (realm of influence) of the kidneys and this stimulates the kidneys, remembering that kidney essence is required to make blood and the kidneys connect directly to the uterus.

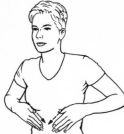

6. Rub the ribs with both palms in a downward direction from the armpits to the centre of the upper abdomen until this area becomes warm to the touch. Then rub from the lower edges of the ribcage to the midpoint of the lower abdomen until this area gets warm.

Lastly, rub from the navel to the pubic bone, in a downward direction only, five to ten times.

Self-massage for premenstrual breast distension and pain

1. Begin by gently massaging any lumps within the breasts for 10 minutes. Then press and knead the centre of the breastbone between the nipples. This is acupuncture point *Shan Zhong* (Conception Vessel 17). It regulates all the qi in the body and especially chest and

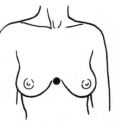

breast qi. It also calms the spirit. Do this 100–200 times.

2. Knead the underarms with the tips of the middle fingers, first one underarm and then the other. Do this 100 times on each side.

3. Push the breasts with both palms simultaneously. Push lightly from every side of the breasts towards the nipples for three to five minutes.

4. Rub the breasts lightly in circles. First rub the circles from the outside to the inside. Then reverse the direction and rub from inside to outside. Do this until the breasts feel warm.

5. Rub the sides of the chest downwards from the armpits to the centre of the upper abdomen in the same way as in the last step of the self-massage for menstrual irregularities (see page 124). Do this until these areas feel warm.

Finally, rub the abdomen in a circle in a clockwise direction around the navel for approximately five minutes.

The key to success with Chinese self-massage therapy is perseverance. Although a single massage may provide some symptomatic relief on that very day, only repeated self-massage day after day can make stable and lasting changes.

FLOWER THERAPY

The beauty of flowers is a wonderful way to bring joy into your life and in Chinese medicine there is actually a practice of flower therapy. Since the beauty of flowers brings most people joy and because joy is the antidote to the other negative emotions of Chinese medicine, flowers can help promote the free and easy flow of qi. Chinese medicine states: 'Joy leads to relaxation (in the flow of qi)' and relaxation is exactly what is required in cases of premenstrual liver depression qi stagnation. As Wu Shi-ji wrote in the Qing dynasty, 'Enjoying flowers can divert a person from their boredom and alleviate suffering caused by the seven effects (emotions).'

There is, however, more to Chinese flower therapy than the beauty of flowers bringing joy. Flower therapy also includes aromatherapy. A number of Chinese medicinals come from plants that have flowers used in bouquets. For instance, chrysanthemum flowers (*Ju Hua*, Flos Chrysanthemi Morifolii) are used to calm the liver and clear depressive heat rising to the upper body. The aroma of chrysanthemums thus also has a health-giving, relaxing and cooling effect on liver depression and depressive heat. Roses (*Mei Gui Hua,* Flos Rosae Rugosae) are used in Chinese medicine to move the qi and quicken the blood. Smelling the fragrance of roses also does the same thing. Other flowers used in Chinese medicine to calm the spirit and relieve stress and irritability are lily, narcissus, lotus flowers, orchids and jasmine. Inhaling the scent of a bouquet of flowers promotes deep breathing and this, in turn, relieves pent-up qi in the chest at the same time as promoting the flow of qi downwards via the lungs.

THREAD MOXIBUSTION

Thread moxibustion refers to burning extremely tiny cones or 'threads' of aged Oriental mugwort directly on top of certain acupuncture points. When done correctly, this is a very simple and effective way of adding yang qi to the body without causing a burn or scar.

To do thread moxibustion, you will need the finest grade Japanese moxa wool. This is available from some of the suppliers listed on pages 152–56, under the name Gold Direct Moxa. Pinch off a very small amount of this loose moxa wool and roll it lightly between the thumb and forefinger to make a very loose, very thin thread of moxa about half the size of a grain of rice. It is important that this thread is not too large or too tightly wrapped.

Next, rub a very thin film of Tiger Balm or Temple of Heaven Balm on the point to be treated. These are camphored Chinese medical salves which are widely available in health food stores. Be sure to apply no more than the thinnest film of salve. If such a Chinese medicated salve is not available, then wipe the point with a tiny amount of vegetable oil or even a small amount of water, something for the moxa thread to stick to. Stand the thread of moxa up on end directly over the point to be treated and light the thread with a burning incense stick.

As the thread burns down towards the skin, you will begin to feel some heat. Immediately remove the burning thread or just press down on it to put it out as soon as you start to feel it warming up. It gets hot very quickly so take great care. It is better to pull the thread off too soon than too late. (If you do burn yourself, apply some *Ching Wan Hong* ointment. This is a Chinese burn salve, which is available at Chinese apothecaries and is truly wonderful for treating all sorts of burns. It should be in every home's medicine cabinet. Lavender essential oil is also very effective.)

Having removed the burning thread or extinguished it, repeat this process. To speed this process up, you can roll a number of threads before starting the treatment. Each time the thread burns down close to the skin, extinguish it before it starts to burn you. If you do this correctly, your skin will get red and hot to the touch but you will not raise a blister. Since everyone's skin is different, the first time you do this, only use three or four threads. Each day, increase this number until you reach 9–12 threads per treatment.

This treatment is especially effective for women in their late 30s and throughout their 40s whose spleen and kidney yang qi has already become weak and insufficient. Since this treatment actually adds yang qi to the body, it fortifies the spleen and invigorates the kidneys, warming yang and boosting the qi. As the stimulus is not that strong at any given treatment, it must be done every day for a number of days. For women who suffer from PMS with pronounced premenstrual fatigue, loose stools, cold hands and feet, low or no libido and lower back or knee pain accompanied by frequent night-time urination which tends to be copious and clear, I recommend beginning this moxibustion just before ovulation, around day 10 in the cycle. It should then be repeated every day until day one of the period and then suspended. It can be done for several months in a row, but should not usually be done

continuously every day throughout
the year. The following three points
should be treated using this
supplementing technique: *Qi Hai*
(Conception Vessel 6), *Guan Yuan*
(Conception Vessel 4) and
Zu San Li (Stomach 36).

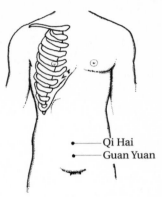

We have already discussed how to
locate *Zu San Li* (see page 115).
However, I recommend visiting a
local professional acupuncturist so
that they can teach you how to do this technique safely and
effectively and to show you how to locate these three points
accurately.

In Chinese medicine, this technique is considered to promote
longevity and good health. It is excellent for those people
whose yang qi has already begun to decline due to the
inevitable ageing process. It should not be done by people
with ascension of hyperactive liver yang, liver fire or
depressive liver heat. It should also always be done by starting
from the topmost point and moving downwards. This is to
prevent leading heat from counterflowing upwards. If there is
any doubt about whether this technique is appropriate for
you, please see a professional practitioner for a diagnosis and
individual recommendation.

CHINESE MEDICAL RESEARCH ON PMS

Considerable research has been done in the People's Republic of China on the effects of acupuncture and Chinese herbal medicine on all aspects of PMS. Usually, this research is in the form of a clinical audit. That means that a group of patients with the same diseases, patterns or major complaints are given the same treatment for a fixed period of time. After this time, the results are examined to see how many patients were cured, how many felt a marked effect, how many felt some effect and how many felt no effect. Until recently, this kind of 'outcome-based' research was not considered credible in the West where, for the last 30 years or so, the double-blind, placebo-controlled comparison study has been considered the 'gold standard'. However, such comparison studies are impossible to design using Chinese medicine and do not, in any case, measure effectiveness in a real-life situation.

Clinical audits, on the other hand, do measure actual clinical satisfaction of real-life patients. Such clinical audits may not exclude the patient's trust and belief in the therapist or the therapy as an important component in the result. However, real life is not as neat and discrete as a controlled laboratory experiment. If the majority of patients are satisfied with the results of a particular treatment and there are no adverse side-effects to that treatment, then that is good enough for the Chinese doctor and, in my experience, that is also good enough for the vast majority of my patients.

Below are abbreviated translations of several recent research articles published in Chinese medical journals on the treatment of premenstrual breast distension and pain, and fibrocystic disease. Many women with premenstrual breast distension and pain also have fibrocystic breasts and, typically, fibrocystic breasts do get worse during the premenstruum. These research articles demonstrate how Chinese medicine treats one of the most common premenstrual complaints. I think that the statistics speak for themselves.

'The Pattern Discrimination Treatment of 90 Cases of Menstrual Movement Breast Distension' by Wang Fa-chang and Wang Qu-an, *Shan Dong Zhong Yi Za Zhi (The Shandong Journal of Chinese Medicine),* **No. 5, 1993**
Menstrual movement, i.e. premenstrual breast distension and pain, is one of the most commonly seen complaints in gynaecology departments. The authors of this clinical audit have treated 90 cases of this condition based on pattern discrimination. Of these 90 women, four were 16–20 years old, 11 were 21–25, 20 were 26–30, 21 were 31–35, 20 were 36–40, five were 41–45, seven were 46–50 and two cases were more than 50 years old. The duration of these women's conditions was from six months to 20 years.

1. Simultaneous liver depression with damp heat pattern
The main symptoms of this pattern are premenstrual chest oppression, heart vexation (anxiety) and easy anger (irritability), breast distension and pain, a dry mouth, vexatious heat of the chest and epigastrium (stomach), lower abdominal aching and pain, possible vaginal itching or excessive, yellow-coloured vaginal discharge, a bowstring, rapid pulse and red tongue with a thin, yellow coating. The treatment principles were to course the liver and resolve depression, clear heat and disinhibit dampness. The formula consisted of a combination of *Dan Zhi Xiao Yao San* (Moutan and Gardenia Rambling Powder), *Yi Huang Tang* (Change Yellow [Discharge] Decoction) and *San Miao San* (Three Wonders Powder) plus Rhizoma Cyperi Rotundi *(Xiang Fu).*

2. Simultaneous liver depression with blood stasis pattern

The main symptoms of this pattern are premenstrual heart vexation (anxiety) and easy anger (irritability), breast distension and pain, occasional nodulation, lower abdominal distension and tenderness, possible scanty, intermittent menstruation, a dark, purplish menstruate containing clots, a bowstring, slippery pulse and a purplish, dark tongue with static spots or patches and a thin, white coating. The treatment principles were to course the liver and resolve depression, quicken the blood, transform stasis and stop pain. The formula consisted of *Dan Zhi Xiao Yao San* (Moutan and Gardenia Rambling Powder) combined with *Tao Hong Si Wu Tang* (Persica and Carthamus Four Materials Decoction) plus Pericarpium Citri Reticulatae Viride *(Qing Pi)*, Rhizoma Corydalis Yanhusuo *(Yan Hu Suo)* and Tuber Curcumae *(Yu Jin)*.

3. Simultaneous liver depression with heart–spleen dual vacuity pattern

The main symptoms of this pattern are premenstrual chest oppression, heart vexation (anxiety) and chaotic thoughts, mild, insidious breast pain or small sensations of distension, heart palpitations, dizziness, loss of sleep, vivid dreams, lack of strength of the entire body, lassitude of the spirit (apathy), diminished appetite, excessive, pasty white vaginal discharge, a bowstring, fine pulse and a pale tongue with teeth marks on its border and a thin, white coating. The treatment principles were to course the liver and resolve depression, fortify the spleen, harmonise the stomach, nourish the heart and quiet the spirit. The formula consisted of *Dan Shen Gui Pi Tang* (Salvia Restore the Spleen Decoction) plus Rhizoma Cyperi Rotundi *(Xiang Fu)* and Tuber Curcumae *(Yu Jin)*.

4. Liver–kidney insufficiency pattern

The main symptoms of this pattern are premenstrual chest oppression, heart vexation (anxiety) and chaotic thoughts, mild, insidious breast pain, dizziness, tinnitus, lower back pain, weakness of the extremities, lack of strength, a deep, bowstring pulse and a pale tongue with a thin coating. The treatment principles were to course the liver and fortify the spleen, supplement and boost the liver and kidneys. The formula consisted of *Dan Zhi Xiao Yao San* (Moutan and Gardenia Rambling Powder) plus Cortex Eucommiae Ulmoidis *(Du Zhong)*, Radix Dipsaci *(Chuan Xu Duan)*, Ramulus Loranthi Seu Visci *(Sang Ji Sheng)*, Cornu Degelatinum Cervi *(Lu Jiao Shuang)*, Fructus Corni Officinalis *(Shan Zhu Yu)* and Semen Cuscutae *(Tu Si Zi)*.

5. Simultaneous liver depression with *chong* and *ren* vacuity cold pattern

The main symptoms of this pattern are premenstrual heart vexation (anxiety) and chaotic thoughts, lassitude of the spirit (apathy), breast distension and pain, insidious lower abdominal pain with a cool sensation, a fine, slow pulse and a pale tongue with a thin, white coating. The treatment principles were to course the liver and resolve depression, cherish the palace (i.e. uterus) and scatter cold. The formula consisted of *Dan Zhi Xiao Yao San* (Moutan and Gardenia Rambling Powder) plus Radix Linderae Strychnifoliae *(Wu Yao)*, Rhizoma Cyperi Rotundi *(Xiang Fu)*, stir-fried Fructus Foeniculi Vulgaris *(Xiao Hui Xiang)* and stir-fried Folium Artemisiae Argyii *(Ai Ye)*.

One course of treatment consisted of three quantities of the above formula. One quantity per day was to be brewed as a tea and administered during the woman's premenstruum. Complete cure was defined as disappearance of such symptoms as premenstrual chest oppression, heart vexation and chaotic thoughts, breast distension and pain, etc., with reduction or disappearance of nodulations and lumps in the breasts within three courses of treatment, i.e. three menstrual cycles. Marked improvement consisted of reduction in such symptoms as premenstrual chest oppression, heart vexation and chaotic thoughts, breast distension and pain, etc., within three courses of treatment. Fair improvement consisted of reduction in the same sorts of symptoms as above in three courses of treatment but recurrence or worsening of these symptoms due to emotional stress. According to these criteria, of the 90 women treated in this study, 57 were cured, 23 were markedly improved, eight experienced fair improvement and two felt no result. Thus the overall improvement rate using this protocol was 97.8 per cent.

'The Treatment of 24 Cases of Fibrocystic Breasts with *Ru Kuai Xiao Tang Jia Wei* (Breast Lump Dispersing Decoction with Added Flavours)' by Hou Jian, *Shan Dong Zhong Yi Za Zhi (The Shandong Journal of Chinese Medicine)*, No. 5, 1993
This clinical audit reports on the treatment of 24 cases of fibrocystic breast disease with *Ru Kuai Xiao Tang Jia Wei* from 1989 to 1991. The ages of the women in this study ranged from 23 to 50 years old, with six cases being between 23 and 30, 15 between 31 and 40 and three between 41 and 50 years of age. The duration of the condition was six months or less in 13 cases, from seven months to one year in five cases, and over one year in six cases. All these women were married. Treatment used a basic formula, which was modified based on pattern discrimination.

1. Liver qi depression and stagnation pattern (13 cases)
The signs and symptoms of this pattern include breast distension and pain that either occurs before the period or becomes worse with the approach of the period, pain and

distension reaching the chest and lateral costal regions, palpable fibrotic tissue and lumps within the breasts but without clearly demarcated borders, lumps that are changeable (i.e. come and go, grow and shrink with the menstrual cycle), a tendency to be overemotional, sighing, chest oppression, a darkish pale tongue with a thin, white coating and a bowstring, fine pulse.

2. Phlegm congelation blood stasis pattern (7 cases)
The signs and symptoms of this pattern include dull breast pain and numbness. However, in prolonged cases, there is piercing pain. In addition, there are soft, pliable, nodular lumps which do not adhere to the underside of the skin. Typically, there is physical fatigue, nausea, vomiting of phlegmy saliva, a gloomy (darkish) tongue with a glossy, slimy coating and a slippery or choppy pulse.

3. *Chong* and *ren* loss of regulation pattern (4 cases)
The signs and symptoms of this pattern include breast heaviness and pain, many breast lumps occurring before, during or after menstruation, emotional tension, agitation and irritability, lower back pain, lack of strength, a pale tongue with a white coating and a soggy or vacuous pulse. This pattern mostly occurs in older women.

Ru Kuai Xiao Tang (the basic formula used in this protocol) consisted of:

15 g	Fructus Trichosanthis Kirlowii *(Gua Lou)*
15 g	Uncooked Concha Ostreae *(Mu Li)*
15 g	Spica Prunellae Vulgaris *(Xia Gu Cao)*
15 g	Thallus Algae *(Kun Bu)*
15 g	Herba Sargassii *(Hai Zao)*
15 g	Radix Salviae Miltiorrhizae *(Dan Shen)*
9 g	Radix Bupleuri *(Chai Hu)*

9 g	Tuber Asparagi Cochinensis *(Tian Men Dong)*
9 g	Rhizoma Sparganii *(San Leng)*
9 g	Rhizoma Curcumae Zedoariae *(E Zhu)*
9 g	Folium Citri (Ju Ye)
9 g	Semen Citri *(Ju He)*
9 g	Rhizoma Pinelliae Ternatae *(Ban Xia)*

The quantities given are decocted in water and make enough for one day's supply, to be administered in two divided doses. Treatment was commenced 15 days before the onset of the period, with 12 days equalling one course of treatment. Administration was discontinued during the period itself.

If the pattern was liver qi depression and stagnation, 9 g Pericarpium Citri Reticulatae Viride *(Qing Pi)* and 9 g Rhizoma Cyperi Rotundi *(Xiang Fu)* were added to move the qi and scatter depression. If the pattern was phlegm congelation and blood stasis, the amounts of Concha Ostreae, Thallus Algae and Radix Salviae Miltiorrhizae were increased up to 30 g each to soften the hard and dispel stasis. If the pattern was *chong* and *ren* loss of regulation, Radix Morindae Officinalis *(Ba Ji Tian)*, Cornu Degelatinum Cervi *(Lu Jiao Shuang)* and Retinervus Luffae Cyclindricae *(Si Gua Luo)* were added to secure the kidneys, rectify the *chong* and free the flow of the network vessels in the breasts.

Complete cure consisted of disappearance of the breast lumps, complete reduction in the aching and pain and no recurrence on follow-up six months later. Some improvement was defined as reduction in the size of the lumps and lessening of the pain and soreness. No improvement meant that there was no change in either the lumps or the pain. Based on these criteria, after one course of treatment, six women were cured and four felt some improvement. After two courses of treatment, three more women were cured and two more got some improvement. After three courses of treatment, three additional women were cured and one more got some improvement. After four courses of treatment, one more was cured, two more improved and two got no result. Therefore, the total number of cases cured was 13, the total number of cases improved was nine, and only two women experienced no result. Thus the overall improvement rate was 91.7 per cent.

The author of this article quotes *Wai Ke Zheng Zong (The True Lineage of External Medicine)* in explaining how this condition comes about:

> Breast aggregation (the traditional Chinese medical name for fibrocystic breasts and breast lumps) consists of nodulations within the breast, their form being like that of an egg. They may be heavy and painful or there may be no pain. The skin over them is not changed. The growth and decline of these lumps may follow (the growth and decline of) joy and anger. They are mostly due to worry and anxiety damaging the spleen and irritation and anger damaging the liver with depression binding producing (nodulation).

'50 Cases Treated for Premenstrual Breast Distension and Pain with *Jie Yu Huo Xue Tang* (Resolve Depression and Quicken the Blood Decoction)' by Gu Si-yun, *Shan Dong Zhong Yi Za Zhi (The Shandong Journal of Chinese Medicine)*, No. 6, 1992

The author of this study begins by saying that premenstrual breast distension is due primarily to liver depression and qi stagnation with subsequent loss of harmony and downbearing of the stomach. Since the breasts are circulated by the liver and stomach channels, qi depression and stagnation affecting these two organs make it difficult for the qi to drain from these channels as they should. A sample of 50 women suffering from premenstrual breast distension and pain were, therefore, treated with the following formula:

15 g   Rhizoma Cyperi Rotundi *(Xiang Fu)*

15 g	Fructus Trichosanthis Kirlowii *(Gua Lou)*
15 g	Radix Salviae Miltiorrhizae *(Dan Shen)*
12 g	Radix Bupleuri *(Chai Hu)*
12 g	Radix Ligustici Wallichii *(Chuan Xiong)*
12 g	Radix Rubrus Paeoniae Lactiflorae *(Chi Shao)*
12 g	Tuber Curcumae *(Yu Jin)*
12 g	Radix Dioscoreae Oppositae *(Shan Yao)*
10 g	Semen Pruni Persicae *(Tao Ren)*
10 g	Pericarpium Citri Reticulatae Viride *(Qing Pi)*
10 g	Folium Citri *(Ju Ye)*
9 g	Flos Carthami Tinctorii *(Hong Hua)*
9 g	Fructus Citri Aurantii *(Zhi Ke)*
6 g	Radix Glycyrrhizae *(Gan Cao)*

If patients suffered from spleen vacuity, Radix Codonopsitis Pilosulae *(Dang Shen)*, Radix Astragali Membranacei *(Huang Qi)*, Rhizoma Atractylodis *(Cang Zhu)*, Rhizoma Atractylodis Macrocephalae *(Bai Zhu)* and Fructus Amomi *(Sha Ren)* were added. If patients suffered from blood vacuity, Radix Angelicae Sinensis *(Dang Gui)*, cooked Radix Rehmanniae *(Shu Di)* and Radix Albus Paeoniae Lactiflorae *(Bai Shao)* were added. If patients suffered from kidney yang vacuity, Cortex Eucommiae Ulmoidis *(Du Zhong)*, Semen Cuscutae *(Tu Si Zi)*, Radix Dipsaci *(Xu Duan)* and Herba Epimedii *(Yin Yang Huo)* were added. If patients suffered from kidney yin vacuity, Rhizoma Anemarrhenae Aspheloidis *(Zhi Mu)*, uncooked Radix Rehmanniae *(Sheng Di)*, Fructus Corni Officinalis *(Shan Zhu Yu)* and Herba Ecliptae Prostratae *(Han Lian Cao)* were added. For liver fire invading the stomach, Fructus Gardeniae Jasminoidis *(Zhi Zi)*, Cortex Radicis Moutan *(Dan Pi)* and Pericarpium Citri Reticulatae *(Chen Pi)* were added. For ascendant hyperactivity of liver yang, Ramulus Uncariae Cum Uncis *(Gou Teng)*, Concha Margaritiferae *(Zhen Zhu Mu)*, Radix Gentianae Scabrae *(Long Dan Cao)* and Flos

Chrysanthemi Morifolii *(Ju Hua)* were added. For yin vacuity and yang hyperactivity, Concha Ostreae *(Mu Li)*, Gelatinum Corii Asini *(E Jiao)*, Tuber Ophiopogonis Japonici *(Mai Dong)* and uncooked Radix Rehmanniae *(Sheng Di)* were added. If there was blood stasis and phlegm congelation, Radix Angelicae Sinensis *(Dang Gui)*, Squama Manitis Pentadactylis *(Chuan Shan Jia)*, Semen Vaccariae Segetalis *(Wang Bu Liu Xing)* and Rhizoma Sparganii *(San Leng)* were added. These ingredients were decocted in water and one quantity of the above herbal medicinals was given per day.

Of the women treated in this study, 20 were between the ages of 15 and 20, 18 were between the ages of 21 and 30 and 12 were 31 or older. The oldest woman was 35. Their condition had lasted from a minimum of six months to a maximum of ten years, with the average being three years. The above treatment was given for three whole months. At the end of that time, 44 cases (88 per cent) experienced complete cure. Another five cases (10 per cent) experienced some improvement, while only a single case (2 per cent) failed to experience any improvement. Thus the overall improvement rate of the patients participating in this study was 98 per cent.

'The Treatment of 128 Cases of Fibrocystic Breasts by Mi Yang, *Hu Nan Zhong Yi Za Zhi (The Hunan Journal of Chinese Medicine)',* No. 1, 1993

This clinical audit describes the treatment of 128 cases of fibrocystic breast disease using a formula called *Shen Xiao Gua Lou San*. In all, 68 cases involved women between the ages of 22–30, 46 cases were aged 31–40 and 14 cases were 41–55 years of age.

The formula used was *Shen Xiao Gua Lou San* (Magically Dispersing Trichosanthes Powder):

15 g   Fructus Trichosanthis Kirlowii *(Quan Gua Lou)*
12 g   Radix Angelicae Sinensis *(Dang Gui)*

10 g   Processed Resina Olibani *(Ru Xiang)*
10 g   Processed Resina Myrrhae *(Mo Yao)*
 6 g   Radix Glycyrrhizae *(Gan Cao)*

These quantities were boiled in 500 ml of water, and produced one day's supply to be taken in two divided doses.

If the symptoms included a disturbed emotional state; chest and lateral costal pain and fullness in the breasts; heart vexation (anxiety) and irritability; premenstrual breast distension and pain; swelling and lumps that felt achy and painful as if heavy; and if pressure caused worsening of the pain, then Radix Bupleuri *(Chai Hu)*, Radix Rubrus Paeoniae Lactiflorae *(Chi Shao)*, Semen Vaccariae Segetalis *(Wang Bu Liu Xing)* and stir-fried Fructus Citri Aurantii *(Zhi Ke)* were added to this formula. If the breast lumps felt stringy or ropey within the breasts or were scattered throughout the breasts; if their nature was pliable but tough; if menstruation was excessive but pale in colour, the limbs were weak and there were dizziness and vertigo, then Radix Astragali Membranacei *(Huang Qi)*, Radix Codonopsitis Pilosulae *(Dang Shen)* and Fructus Liquidambaris Taiwaniae *(Lu Lu Tong)* were added. If the breasts were swollen and painful and scorching hot, the tongue was red with a thin, yellow coating and the pulse was bowstring and rapid, Flos Lonicerae Japonicae *(Jin Yin Hua)*, Fructus Forsythiae Suspensae *(Lian Qiao)* and Herba Taraxaci Mongolici Cum Radice *(Pu Gong Ying)* were added. If the breast lumps were comparatively firm but not hard, tender when pressed and shifted position when pushed, blast-fried Squama Manitis Pentadactylis *(Chuan Shan Jia)*, Spina Gleditschiae Chinensis *(Zao Jiao Ci)*, Rhizoma Sparganii *(San Leng)* and Rhizoma Curcumae Zedoariae *(E Zhu)* were added.

Treatment lasted between 30 and 180 days, with the average being 50 days. Complete cure was defined as disappearance of the lumps. Marked improvement was defined as reduction in the pain and aching and decrease in the size of the lumps. No result was defined as no diminution in the pain or aching and no decrease in the size of the lumps. Based on these criteria, 80 cases (62.5 per cent) of the women in this study experienced complete cure; 42 (32.81 per cent) experienced marked improvement; and six cases got no result. Thus the overall improvement rate was 95.31 per cent.

'The Pattern Discrimination Treatment of 100 Cases of Fibrocystic Breasts by Fang Jian-ping, *Jiang Su Zhong Yi (Jiangsu Chinese Medicine)*', No. 2, 1993

This research report describes the treatment of 100 cases of fibrocystic breast disease based on treating according to a discrimination of patterns. Four patients were between the ages of 15 and 20; 25 were 21–30; 54 were 31–40; and there were 17 cases between 41 and 50 years of age. Ten were unmarried and 90 were married.

1. Liver depression qi stagnation pattern (45 cases)

The lumps within these women's breasts were as large as date stones. They also presented with emotional tension, heart vexation (anxiety) and irritability. The women's menstruation was not easy and there was premenstrual breast heaviness and discomfort, distension and pain. The tongue fur was thin, white or yellow and the pulse was bowstring. The therapeutic principles were to course the liver and resolve depression, move the qi and scatter nodulation. The formula used was *Xiao Yao San Jia Jian* (Rambling Powder with Additions and Subtractions):

10 g   Radix Albus Paeoniae Lactiflorae *(Bai Shao)*
10 g   Sclerotium Poriae Cocos *(Fu Ling)*
10 g   Radix Angelicae Sinensis *(Dang Gui)*
10 g   Herba Taraxaci Mongolici Cum Radice *(Pu Gong Ying)*

10 g	Pericarpium Trichosanthis Kirlowii *(Gua Lou Pi)*
10 g	Pericarpium Citri Reticulatae Viride *(Qing Pi)*
10 g	Rhizoma Atractylodis Macrocephalae *(Bai Zhu)*
10 g	Semen Citri *(Ju He)*
6 g	Processed Squama Manitis Pentadactylis *(Chuan Shan Jia)*
5 g	Vinegar-fried Radix Bupleuri *(Chai Hu)*
5 g	Stir-fried Fructus Gardeniae Jasminoidis *(Shan Zhi Zi)*
3 g	Roasted Rhizoma Zingiberis *(Wei Jiang)*
3 g	Radix Glycyrrhizae *(Gan Cao)*

2. Liver depression qi vacuity pattern (23 cases)

These women's lumps were movable, and divided and scattered or blended into the rest of the tissue and so were not easily discernible. Their facial colour was sallow white and they had dizziness and vertigo, were exhausted and lacked strength. Their menses were excessive but pale in colour and their tongues were pale with a thin, white coating. Their pulses were soggy and fine. The therapeutic principles for this presentation were to course the liver and scatter nodulation, boost the qi and nourish the blood. The formula used was *Si Wu Tang Jia Jian* (Four Materials Decoction with Additions and Subtractions):

10 g	Cooked Radix Rehmanniae *(Shu Di)*
10 g	Radix Angelicae Sinensis *(Dang Gui)*
10 g	Radix Albus Paeoniae Lactiflorae *(Bai Shao)*
10 g	Radix Astragali Membranacei *(Huang Qi)*
10 g	Sclerotium Poriae Cocos *(Fu Ling)*
10 g	Tuber Curcumae *(Yu Jin)*
10 g	Herba Taraxaci Mongolici Cum Radice *(Pu Gong Ying)*
10 g	Fructus Liquidambaris Taiwaniae *(Lu Lu Tong)*
6 g	Processed Squama Manitis Pentadactylis *(Chuan Shan Jia)*
5 g	Radix Ligustici Wallichii *(Chuan Xiong)*

5 g   Cornu Degelatinum Cervi *(Lu Jiao Shuang)*
3 g   Vinegar-fried Radix Bupleuri *(Chai Hu)*

3. Liver depression phlegm nodulation pattern (18 cases)

These women's lumps were shaped like flat discs or lobes. Their chests, lateral costal regions and stomachs were oppressed and distended and they suffered from dizziness, a slightly bitter taste in the mouth, abnormal appetite, clots within their menstrual flow, possible loose stools, a pale tongue with a white, slimy coating and a slippery pulse. The therapeutic principles in this case were to course the liver and flush phlegm, soften the hard and scatter nodulation. The formula used was *Lou Feng Fang Tang Jia Jian* (Nidus Vespae Decoction with Additions and Subtractions):

25 g   Spica Prunellae Vulgaris *(Xia Gu Cao)*
12 g   Processed Rhizoma Cyperi Rotundi *(Xiang Fu)*
10 g   Tuber Curcumae *(Yu Jin)*
10 g   Pericarpium Citri Reticulatae Viride *(Qing Pi)*
10 g   Bulbus Fritillariae Thunbergii *(Bei Mu)*
10 g   Folium Citri *(Ju Ye)*
 6 g   Nidus Vespae *(Lou Feng Fang)*
 6 g   Bulbus Cremastrae *(Shan Ci Gu)*
 6 g   Processed Squama Manitis Pentadactylis *(Chuan Shan Jia)*
 6 g   Radix Bupleuri *(Chai Hu)*

4. Qi stagnation blood stasis pattern (14 cases)

These women's lumps were round and comparatively hard. They might also be shaped like discs or lobes. There was aching and pain and they were tender if pressed. These lumps had been soft or slippery but had changed. There were clots in these women's menstruate and its colour was purplish and dark. Their tongues were purple in colour or had purple patches. Their pulses were fine and bowstring. The therapeutic principles in this case were to quicken the blood and dispel stasis, soften the hard and scatter nodulation (disperse the lumps). The formula used was *Jie Yu Ruan Jian Tang* (Resolve Depression and Soften the Hard Decoction):

12 g	Herba Taraxaci Mongolici Cum Radice *(Pu Gong Ying)*
10 g	Radix Angelicae Sinensis *(Dang Gui)*
10 g	Mix-fried Radix Rubrus Paeoniae Lactiflorae *(Chi Shao)*
10 g	Fructus Tribuli Terrestris *(Bai Ji Li)*
10 g	Thallus Algae *(Kun Bu)*
10 g	Herba Sargassii *(Hai Zao)*
10 g	Cornu Degelatinum Cervi *(Lu Jiao Shuang)*
10 g	Radix Salviae Miltiorrhizae *(Dan Shen)*
10 g	Fructus Crataegi *(Shan Zha)*
6 g	Processed Rhizoma Cyperi Rotundi *(Xiang Fu)*
6 g	Processed Squama Manitis Pentadactylis *(Chuan Shan Jia)*
6 g	Tuber Curcumae *(Yu Jin)*
5 g	Radix Ligustici Wallichii *(Chuan Xiong)*
5 g	Radix Bupleuri *(Chai Hu)*
5 g	Pericarpium Citri Reticulatae Viride *(Qing Pi)*
5 g	Bulbus Cremastrae *(Shan Ci Gu)*

The above medicinals were administered in decoction internally. At the same time, *Xiao Yan Gao* (Disperse Inflammation Plaster) plus *Ru Kuai San* (Breast Lump Powder) were applied externally, over the lumps.

The criteria for success using these protocols were as follows: complete cure was defined as disappearance of the lumps, disappearance of the breast pain and discontinuance of the medicinals after three months. Marked improvement was defined as reduction of the size of the lumps by half and disappearance of the breast pain. Some improvement was defined as reduction of the size of the lumps by less than half and reduction in the breast pain. No result was defined as no reduction in the size of the breast lumps.

Of those suffering from liver depression qi stagnation, 37 experienced complete cure; six, marked improvement; and two, some improvement. Of those suffering from liver depression qi vacuity, 16 experienced complete cure; five, marked improvement; and two, some improvement. Of those suffering from qi depression phlegm nodulation, 11 experienced complete cure; five, marked improvement; one, some improvement; and one, no result. Of those suffering from qi stagnation blood stasis, eight experienced complete cure; three, marked improvement; one, some improvement; and two, no result. Therefore, the total number of complete cures was 72; marked improvement, 19; some improvement, six; and no result, three. Thus the overall improvement rate was 97 per cent.

FINDING A PRACTITIONER OF CHINESE MEDICINE

C hinese medicine is one of the fastest growing holistic health care systems in the West today. In the UK there are at least ten colleges offering a professional training courses in acupuncture, moxibustion, Chinese herbal medicine and Chinese medical massage; some offer a university degree. In addition, many of the graduates of these courses have done postgraduate studies at colleges and hospitals in China, Taiwan, Hong Kong and Japan. A growing number of trained Oriental medical practitioners have emigrated from China, Japan and Korea to practice acupuncture and Chinese herbal medicine in the West.

Chinese medicine, including acupuncture, is a discrete and independent health care profession. It is not simply a technique that can easily be added to the array of techniques of some other health care profession. The study of Chinese medicine, acupuncture and Chinese herbs is as rigorous as is the study of allopathic, chiropractic, naturopathic or homoeopathic medicine. Previous training in any one of these other systems does not automatically confer competence or knowledge in Chinese medicine. In order to get the full benefits and ensure the safety of Chinese medicine, it is best to seek out professionally trained and qualified practitioners.

When seeking a qualified and knowledgeable practitioner, personal recommendations are often the best method. It is essential to work with a practitioner who communicates effectively enough for the patient to feel understood. Here are some questions you might ask when selecting a practitioner:

- Where did you qualify and are you a member of the appropriate professional body?

- What is your experience in treating my condition?
- Do you use disposable needles?
- How often will I need to see you and for how many visits?
- How much do you charge?

Many practitioners will be happy to talk on the phone or offer a short introductory consultation so that you can assess whether you will feel comfortable working with them.

Below is a list of professional bodies for Chinese medicine in the UK. I have included information on shiatsu practitioners as it can be a very effective therapy to treat headaches.

Acupuncture
The British Acupuncture Council
63 Jeddo Road
London
W12 9HQ
Tel: 020 8735 0400
Fax: 020 8735 0404
E-mail: infor@acupuncture.org.uk
Website: www.acupuncture.org.uk

Members have the initials: MBAcC.

Chinese herbal medicine
The Register of Chinese Herbal Medicine
PO Box 400
Wembley
Middlesex
HA9 9NZ
Tel/fax: 07000 790332
Website: www.rchm.co.uk

Members have the initials: MRCHM.

Japanese herbal medicine
The Kanpo Association
9a Ingatestone Road
Brentwood
Essex
CM15 8AP
Tel: 01277 260080

Members have the initials: KANPO.
Members of the Kanpo Association are not bound by a code of
ethics and practice or covered by insurance unless they also
belong to another professional body. Most practitioners of
kanpo belong to one of the three other professional bodies.

Shiatsu
The Shiatsu Society UK
Barber House
Storeys Bar Road
Fengate
Peterborough
PE1 5YS
Tel: 01733 758341
E-mail: shiatsu@graphic-scan.co.uk

Members have the initials: MRSS.

Relevant bodies in other English-speaking countries are:

**Australian Acupuncture and Chinese Medical Association
(AACMA)**
PO Box 5142
West End
Brisbane
Queensland
Australia 4101

Tel: +07 3846 5866
Fax: +07 3846 5276
Free Call: 1800 025 334
E-mail: aaca@eis.net.au
Website: http://www2.eis.net.au/-aaca

**The International Institute of Chinese Medicine
and Acupuncture**
PO Box 2246
19 Av Disandt-Fresnaye
Cape Town 8000
South Africa
Tel: 27 21 434 1654

LEARNING MORE ABOUT CHINESE MEDICINE

Acupuncture and Chinese medicine in general

The Web That Has No Weaver: Understanding Chinese Medicine, Ted Kaptchuk, Congdon and Weed, New York, 1983
This is the best overall introduction to Chinese medicine for the serious lay reader. It has been a standard since it was first published over a dozen years ago and it has yet to be replaced.

Clinical Handbook of Chinese Prepared Medicine, Chun-han Zhu, Paradigm Publications, Brookline, Massachusetts, 1989
This book is an excellent reference text for Chinese prepared or patent medicines. It uses a professionally accurate, standard translation so the terminology is similar to that used in this book. It is beautifully designed and laid out and is easy to use. This is most definitely my first choice of books on Chinese patent medicines.

Chinese Medicine: Acupuncture, Herbal Remedies, Nutrition, Qui Gong and Meditation, Tom Williams, Element Health Essentials
This is a good basic introduction to the whole field of Chinese medicine for the layperson.

Acupuncture, Peter Mole, Element Books
A simple and clear introduction to acupuncture for the layperson.

A Guide to Acupuncture, Peter Firebrace and Sandra Hill, Constable Books
A comprehensive introduction to acupuncture for the layperson with some illustrations and photographs.

Between Heaven and Earth: A Guide to Chinese Medicine, Harriet Beinfield and Efrem Corngold, Ballantine Books, New York
This book is particularly good with regard to the more psychological and emotional aspects of Chinese medicine and has a good introduction to herbal medicine for the layperson.

Acupuncture in Practice, Hugh McPherson and Ted Kaptchuk (eds), Churchill Livingstone
This is a book of case histories from the West; it illustrates the wide variety of styles and methods of practice of acupuncture by many well-known practitioners.

Chinese Herbal Medicine, A Practical Guide to the Healing Powers of Herbs, Dr Guang Xu, Vermillion
A good introduction to Chinese herbal medicine.

Japanese Acupuncture, A Clinical Guide, Stephen Birch and Junko Ida, Paradigm Publications
This book gives very good, clear details on moxibustion but is aimed at practitioner level.

Menopause, A Second Spring: Making a Smooth Transition with Chinese Medicine, Honiara Lee Wolfe, Blue Poppy Press, Boulder, Colorado

Chinese dietary therapy
Healing with Wholefoods, Oriental Traditions and Modern Nutrition, Paul Pritchard, North Atlantic Books
A comprehensive source book for both the layperson and the professional.

Helping Ourselves: A Guide to the Traditional Chinese Food Energetics, Daverick Legget, Meridian Press
This book is designed for ease of use with its clear layout and wallcharts.

Chinese Medical Wines and Elixirs, Bob Flaws, Blue Poppy Press, Boulder, Colorado

The Book of Jook: Chinese Medical Porridges: A Healthy Alternative to the Typical Western Breakfast, Bob Flaws, Blue Poppy Press, Boulder, Colorado

Chinese Medicinal Teas: Simple, Proven, Folk Formulas for Common Diseases and Promoting Health, Zong Xiao-fan and Gary Liscum, Blue Poppy Press, Boulder, Colorado

Asian psychology and psychotherapy

The Quiet Therapies: Japanese Pathways to Personal Growth, David K. Reynolds, University of Hawaii Press, Honolulu, 1987
This book is a good introduction to Japanese forms of psychotherapy based on a practical, rather than analytical approach. It also discusses the psychotherapeutic benefits of deep relaxation.
Also by the same author:
Playing Ball on Running Water
Even in Winter the Ice Doesn't Melt

Tibetan Buddhist Medicine and Psychiatry: The Diamond Healing, Terry Clifford, Samuel Weiser Inc., York Beach, ME, 1984
This book explains the Tibetan Buddhist approach to the diagnosis and treatment of mental–emotional disorders. Although Tibetan medicine is not exactly the same as Chinese medicine, they are historically related and many of the insights of Tibetan medicine in terms of psychological disorders are very profound and effective.

SUPPLIERS OF CHINESE HERBAL MEDICINES AND SPECIALIST PRODUCTS

In the UK, it is not possible to buy Chinese herbal medicines over the counter: you will need a prescription from a qualified Chinese herbalist. Some acupuncturists are able to prescribe traditional remedies or 'patents'. The suppliers we have listed here are members of CMAS – The Chinese Medicine Association of Suppliers. CMAS is a professional organisation that acts as a self-regulatory body to lobby in the interests of its members within the bounds of public safety. All members are subject to a code of practice. CMAS is a rapidly growing organisation so it may have more members since this list was completed.

Many of the members of CMAS have an excellent supply of books and other products relating to Chinese medicine and acupuncture. Most, if not all, suppliers have a mail-order service.

This list is by no means exhaustive. There are many other suppliers of acupuncture products and many shops that sell Chinese herbs. The acupuncture product suppliers are a good source should you wish to buy the Japanese pure moxa mentioned in the chapter on home remedies. Please note that the Chinese herbal medicine shops one sees on many high streets may not be regulated.

Acumedic (range of products and books)
101–5 Camden High Street
London
NW1 7JN
Tel: 0171 388 5783
Fax: 0171 387 5766

Beijing Tong Ren Tang (herbal products)
124 Shaftesbury Avenue
London
W1V 7DJ
Tel: 0171 287 0098
Fax: 0171 287 0068

China Medica (herbal products)
25 Lonsdale Close
London
SE9 4HF
Tel: 0181 857 9777
Fax: 0181 480 2020

Chinese Medical Centre (herbal products)
179 South Street
Romford
Essex
RM1 1PS
Tel: 01708 756363
Fax: 01708 703015

East West Herbs (range of products and books)
Langston Priory Mews
Kingham
Oxfordshire
OX7 6UP
Tel: 01608 658862
Fax: 01608 658816
E-mail: robert@eastwestherbs.co.uk

Great Wall (herbal products)
Unit 27
Riverside Works
Hertford Road
Barking
Essex
IG11 8BN
Tel: 0181 591 6896
Fax: 0181 591 6891

Harmony Medical Distribution (range of products)
629 High Road
Leytonstone
London
E11 4PA
Tel: 0181 518 7337
Fax: 0181 556 5038
E-mail: harmony@tcm.org.uk

Lotus (herbal products)
Priorsfield Priory
Forest Row
Sussex
RH18 5HR
Tel: 01342 823053
Fax: 01342 826027
E-mail: user@lotus.u-net.com

Mayway UK (herbal products)
43 Waterside Trading Centre
Trumpers Way
Hanwell
Middlesex
Tel: 0181 893 6873
Fax: 0181 893 6874

Naturally Chinese (range of products)
PO Box 4584
Kiln Farm
Milton Keynes
Bucks
MK13 9BT
Tel: 0151 571 0407

Number One Herb Co. (herbal products)
36 Bankhurst Road
Catford
London
SE6 4XN
Tel: 0181 690 4840
Fax: 0181 690 4840
E-mail: jarrah@vossnet.co.uk

Oxford Medical Supplies (range of products)
Units 11 & 12
Horcott Industrial Estate
Fairford
Gloucestershire
GL7 4LX
Tel: 0800 975 8000
Fax: 0800 975 8111
E-mail: oxfordms@demon.co.uk

Shizhen TCM UK Ltd (herbal products)
50 Sandy Lane
Chorlton
Manchester
M21
Tel: 0161 881 0088
Fax: 0161 881 0888

Tian Tiao Ltd (herbal products)
85 Sullivan Way
Elstree
Herts
WD6 3DG
Tel: 0181 953 2320
Fax: 0181 953 3338

CHINESE MEDICAL GLOSSARY

Chinese medicine is a system unto itself. Its technical terms are uniquely its own and cannot be reduced to the definitions of Western medicine without destroying the very fabric and logic of Chinese medicine. Ultimately, because Chinese medicine was created in the Chinese language, Chinese medicine is really only understood in that language. Nevertheless, we Westerners trying to understand Chinese medicine must translate the technical terms of Chinese medicine into English words. If some of these technical translations sound peculiar at first and their meaning is not immediately clear, this is because no equivalent concepts exist in everyday English.

In the past, some Western authors have erroneously translated technical Chinese medical terms using Western medical or at least quasi-scientific words in an attempt to make this system more acceptable to Western audiences. For instance, the words 'tonify' and 'sedate' are commonly seen in the Western Chinese medical literature even though, in the case of 'sedate', its meaning is completely opposite to the Chinese understanding of the word *xie*. *Xie* means to drain off something that has pooled and accumulated. That accumulation is seen as something excess, which should not be lingering where it is. Because it is accumulating somewhere where it shouldn't be, it is impeding and obstructing whatever should be moving to and through that area. The word 'sedate' comes from the Latin word *sedere*, to sit, so to sedate means to make something sit still. However, the Chinese word *xie* means draining off that which is sitting somewhere erroneously. Therefore, to think that one is going to sedate what is already sitting is a great mistake in understanding the clinical implication and application of this technical term.

Hence, in order to preserve the integrity of this system while still making it intelligible to English language readers, we have appended the following glossary of Chinese medical technical terms. The terms themselves are based on Nigel Wiseman's *English–Chinese Chinese–English Dictionary of Chinese Medicine* (see page 168). Dr Wiseman is, I believe, the greatest Western scholar in terms of the translation of Chinese medicine into English. Although Wiseman's terms may be awkward sounding at first, they convey most accurately the Chinese understanding and logic of these terms.

Acquired essence: Essence manufactured out of the surplus of qi and blood in turn created out of the refined essence of food and drink

Acupoints: Those places on the channels and network vessels where qi and blood tend to collect in denser concentrations and thus those places where the qi and blood in the channels are especially available for manipulation

Acupuncture: The regulation of qi flow by the stimulation of certain points located on the channels and network vessels achieved mainly by insertion of fine needles into these points

Aromatherapy: Using various scents and smells to treat and prevent disease

Ascendant hyperactivity of liver yang: Out of control, upward counterflow of liver yang due to there being insufficient yin to hold it down in the lower part of the body

Astringent: Constricting and containing, keeping in rather than letting go

Blood: The red-coloured fluids that flow in the vessels and nourish and construct the tissues of the body

Blood stasis: Also called dead blood, malign blood and dry blood, blood stasis is blood that is no longer moving through the vessels as it should. Instead it is precipitated in the vessels like silt in a river. It then obstructs the free flow of the blood in the vessels and also impedes the production of new or fresh blood

Blood vacuity: Insufficient blood manifesting in diminished nourishment, construction and moistening of body tissues

Bowels: The hollow yang organs of Chinese medicine

Bowstring: A quality of pulse that feels taut; *see* **Pulse**

Burners: Areas of the abdomen, known as the upper, middle and lower burners, that act as a kind of crucible, known as the triple burner, in which the vital energies are transformed and created by heat

Central qi: Also called the middle qi, this is synonymous with the spleen–stomach qi

Channels: The main routes for the distribution of qi and blood, but mainly qi

Chest oppression: A feeling of tightness and stuffiness in the chest. As a reaction to this feeling, the person will often sigh in an attempt to inhale fresh air and exhale the pent-up stale air

***Chong* and *ren*:** Two of the eight extraordinary vessels that act as reservoirs for all the other channels and vessels of the body. These two govern women's menstruation, reproduction and lactation in particular.

Choppy: A choppy pulse is a fine, somewhat slow pulse which tends to speed up and slow down (often with the breathing) but does not necessarily skip any beats; *see* **Pulse**

Clear: The pure or clear part of ingested food and drink that is then turned into qi and blood

Cold: A pathogenic factor that can invade the body. May combine with wind to form wind cold invasion. Can also be produced as a weakness of internal physiological processes. Cold may be scattered, i.e. broken up and released from the body through treatment.

Constructive qi: The qi that flows through the channels and nourishes and constructs the internal organs and body tissues

Counterflow: An erroneous flow of qi, usually upwards but sometimes horizontally as well

Coursing the liver: Encouraging the correct functioning of the liver viscera with regard to the flow of qi throughout the body

Damp heat: A combination of accumulated dampness mixed with pathological heat often associated with sores, abnormal vaginal discharges and some types of menstrual and body pain

Dampness: A pathological accumulation of body fluids, such as phlegm

Deep: A pulse quality; *see* **Pulse**

Defensive qi: The yang qi that protects the exterior of the body from invasion by wind, cold, heat or dampness

Depression: Stagnation and lack of movement, as in liver depression qi stagnation

Depressive heat: Heat due to enduring or severe qi stagnation, which then transforms into heat

Drain: To drain off or away some pathological qi or substance from where it is replete or excess

Essence: A stored, very potent form of substance and qi, usually yin when compared to yang qi, but can be transformed into yang qi

Evils: Pathogens that enter the body

External causes of disease: The six environmental excesses

Fine: A pulse quality; *see* **Pulse**

Fire (life gate fire, fire effulgence): A pathogenic factor that is usually created within the body

Heart vexation: An irritating, possibly dry, hot sensation in the chest in front of the heart; also anxiety

Heat toxins: A particularly virulent and concentrated type of pathological heat often associated with purulence (i.e. pus formation), sores and sometimes, but not always, malignancies

Heliotherapy: Exposure of the body to sunlight in order to treat and prevent disease

Hydrotherapy: Using various baths and water applications to treat and prevent disease

Impediment: A hindrance to the free flow of the qi and blood typically manifesting as pain and restriction in the range of movement of a joint or extremity

Internal causes of disease: The seven effects or emotions, namely anger, joy (or excitement), sorrow, thought, fear, melancholy and fright

Lassitude of the spirit: A listless or apathetic effect or emotional demeanour due to obvious fatigue of the mind and body

Life gate fire: Another name for kidney yang or kidney fire, seen as the ultimate source of yang qi in the body

Mansion: Realm of influence of one of the viscera

Moxibustion: Burning the herb Artemisia Argyium on, over or near acupuncture points in order to add yang qi, to warm cold, or promote the movement of the qi and blood

Network vessels: Small vessels that form a net-like web ensuring the flow of qi and blood to all body tissues

Pattern discrimination: Basis for diagnosis in TCM. A pattern is determined by the signs and symptoms and by observations of the individual patient's condition

Phlegm: A pathological accumulation of phlegm or mucus congealed from dampness or body fluids

Portals: Also called orifices, the openings of the sensory organs and the opening of the heart through which the spirit makes contact with the world outside

Pulse: Taking the pulse forms an important part of Chinese medical diagnosis. It is taken from the radial artery at both wrists and there are six different pulse positions at each wrist, giving information about the different viscera, bowels and channels. There are 28 types of pulse quality in classic Chinese medicine, including deep, empty, fine, slippery, etc.

Qi: Activity, function, that which moves, transforms, defends, restrains and warms

Qi mechanism: The process of transforming yin substance controlled and promoted by the qi, largely synonymous with the process of digestion

Qi vacuity: Insufficient qi manifesting in diminished movement, transformation and function

Rectifying qi: Making the qi move, particularly in the right direction

Repletion: Excess or fullness, almost always pathological

Resolve the exterior: Release and clear the pathogens from the outer layers of the body where its primary mechanisms are located.

Slippery: A pulse quality; *see* **Pulse**

Soggy: A pulse quality; *see* **Pulse**

Spirit: The accumulation of qi in the heart that manifests as consciousness, sensory awareness and mental–emotional function

Stagnation: Non-movement of the qi, lack of free flow, constraint

Supplement: To add to or augment, as in supplementing the qi, blood, yin, or yang

Turbid: The yin, impure, turbid part of food and drink that is sent downwards to be excreted as waste

Vacuity: Emptiness or insufficiency, typically of qi, blood, yin, or yang

Vacuity cold: Obvious signs and symptoms of cold due to a lack or insufficiency of yang qi

Vacuity heat: Heat due to hyperactive yang in turn due to insufficient controlling yin

Vessels: The main routes for the distribution of qi and blood, but mainly blood

Viscera: The solid yin organs of Chinese medicine

Wind: An unseen pathogen that invades the body's defences. May combine with cold to form wind cold invasion.

Yang: In the body, function, movement, activity and transformation

Yang vacuity: Insufficient warming and transforming function giving rise to symptoms of cold in the body

Yin: In the body, substance and nourishment

Yin vacuity: Insufficient yin substance necessary to nourish, control and counterbalance yang activity

BIBLIOGRAPHY

CHINESE LANGUAGE SOURCES

'A Review of the Chinese Medical Literature on Climacteric Syndrome', Yao Shi-an, *Zhong Yi Za Zhi (Journal of Chinese Medicine)*, No. 2, 1994

'A Study on the Treatment of Primary Dysmenorrhoea with *Jia Wei Mo Jie Tang* (Added Flavours Myrrh and Dragon's Blood Decoction) and Its Effect on Prostaglandins and Related Factors', Zhu Nan-sun *et al.*, *Zhong Yi Za Zhi (Journal of Chinese Medicine*, No. 2, 1994

Bai Ling Fu Ke (Bai-ling's Gynaecology), Han Bai-ling, Heilong-jiang People's Press, Harbin, 1983

Cheng Dan An Zhen Jiu Xuan Ji (Cheng Dan An's Selected Acupuncture and Moxibustion Works), ed. Cheng Wei-fen *et al.*, Shanghai Science and Technology Press, Shanghai, 1986

Chu Zhen Zhi Liao Xue (A Study of Acupuncture Treatment), Li Zhong-yu, Sichuan Science and Technology Press, Chengdu, 1990

'Clinical Experiences in the Treatment of 120 Cases of Mammary Neoplasia with *Ru Tong Ling* (Breast Pain Efficacious [Remedy])', Ye Xiu-min and Zhang Geng-yang, *Tian Jin Zhong Yi (Tianjin Chinese Medicine)*, No. 3, 1994

Dong Yuan Yi Ji (Dong-yuan's Collected Medical Works), ed. Bao Zheng-fei *et al.*, People's Health and Hygiene Press, Beijing, 1993

'Experiences in the Treatment of Chronic Fibrocystic Breast Disease', Yang Hui-an, *Tian Jin Zhong Yi (Tianjin Chinese Medicine)*, No. 6, 1993

Fu Ke Bing (Gynaecological Diseases), California Certified Acupuncturists Association, Oakland, California 1988.

Fu Ke Bing Liang Fang (Fine Formulae for Gynaecological Diseases), He Yuan-lin and Jiang Chang-yun, Yunnan University Press, Chongqing, 1991

Fu Ke Lin Chuan Jing Hua (The Clinical Efflorescence of Gynaecology), Wang Bu-ru and Wang Qi-ming, Sichuan Science and Technology Press, Chengdu, 1989

Fu Ke San Bai Zheng (300 Gynaecological Conditions), Liu Lan-fang and Liu Dian-gong, Jiangxi Science and Technology Press, 1989

Fu Ke Yu Chi (The Jade Ruler of Gynaecology), Shen Jin-ao, Shanghai Science and Technology Press, Shanghai, 1983

Fu Ke Zheng Zhi (Gynaecological Patterns and Treatments), Sun Jiu-ling, Hebei People's Press, 1983

Fu Qing Zhu Nu Ke (Fu Qing-zhu's Gynaecology), Fu Qing-zhu, Shanghai People's Press, Shanghai, 1979; available in English, trans. Yang Shou-zhong and Liu Da-wei, Blue Poppy Press, Boulder, Colorado, 1992

Fu Ren Da Quan Liang Fang (A Great Compendium of Fine Formulae for Women), Chen Ze-ming, People's Government Press, Beijing, 1985

Gu Qin Fu Ke Zhen Jiu Miao Fa Da Cheng (A Great Compendium of Ancient and Modern Acupuncture and Moxibustion Miraculous Methods for Gynaecology), Liu Ji, Chinese National Chinese Medicine and Medicinals Press, Beijing, 1993

Han Ying Chang Yong Yi Xue Ci Hui (Chinese–English Glossary of Commonly Used Medical Terms), Huang Xiao-kai, People's Health and Hygiene Press, Beijing, 1982

He Zi Huai Nu Ke Jing Yan Ji (A Collection of He Zi-huai's Experiences in Gynaecology), Chen Shao-chun and Lu Zhi (eds), Zhejiang Science and Technology Press, 1982

'Lu De-ming's Experiences Treating Mammary Hyperplasia Disease', Hua-fa, *Shang Hai Zhong Yi Yao Za Zhi (Shanghai Journal of Chinese Medicine and Medicinals)*, No. 2, 1994

Nan Nu Bing Mi Yan Liang Fang (Secret, Proven, Fine Formulae for Men's and Women's Disease), Du Jie-hui, Beijing Science and Technology Press, Beijing, 1991

Nu Bing Wai Zhi Liang Fang Miao Fa (Fine Formulae and Miraculous Methods for the External Treatment of Women's Diseases), Wang Jin-quan and Cai Yu-hua, Chinese National Chinese Medicine and Medicinals Press, Beijing, 1993

Nu Ke Bai Wen (100 Questions on Gynaecology), Qi Chong-fu, Shanghai Ancient Chinese Medical Books Press, Shanghai, 1983

Nu Ke Ji Yao (The Collected Essentials of Gynaecology), Yu Yao-feng, People's Government Press, Beijing, 1988

Nu Ke Jing Wei (Profundities from the Gynaecological Classics), Lu Guo-zhi and Song Shu-de, Shanxi Science and Technology Press, Xian, 1989

Nu Ke Mi Jue Da Quan (A Compendium of Secrets of Success in Gynaecology), Chen Liang-fang, Beijing Daily Press, Beijing, 1989

Nu Ke Xian Fang (Immortal Formulae in Gynaecology), Fu Shan, a.k.a. Fu Qing-zhu, Ancient Chinese Medical Book Press, Beijing, 1989

Nu Ke Yao Zhi (The Essentials of Gynaecology), Yu Yo-yuan, Fujian Science and Technology Press, Fuzhou, 1982

Nu Ke Zong Yao (Assembled Essentials of Gynaecology), Zhang Shou-qian, Hunan Science and Technology Press, Changsha, 1985

Ru Fang Ji Huan (Breast Diseases and Sufferings), Qiu Si-kang, People's Health and Hygiene Press, Beijing, 1985

Shang Hai Lao Zhong Yi Jing Yan Xuan Bian (A Selected Compilation of Shanghai Old Doctors' Experiences), Shanghai Science and Technology Press, Shanghai, 1984

Shi Yong Zhen Jiu Tui Na Zhi Liao Xue (A Study of Practical Acupuncture, Moxibustion and Tui Na Treatments), Xia Zhi-ping, Shanghai College of Chinese Medicine Press, Shanghai, 1990

Shi Yong Zhong Xi Yi Jie He Fu Chan Ke Zheng Zhi (Proven Treatments in Practical Integrated Chinese–Western Obstetrics and Gynaecology), Guo Yuan, Shanxi People's Press, Xian, 1984

Tan Zheng Lun (Treatise on Phlegm Conditions), Hou Tian-yin and Wang Chun-hua, People's Army Press, Beijing, 1989

'The Pattern Discrimination Treatment of 90 Cases of Menstrual Movement Breast Distension', Wang Fa-chang and Wang Qu-an, *Shan Dong Zhong Yi Za Zhi (Shandong Journal of Chinese Medicine)*, No. 5, 1993

'The Pattern Discrimination Treatment of 100 Cases of Mammary Hyperplasia', Fang Jian-ping, *Jiang Su Zhong Yi (Jiangsu Chinese Medicine)*, No. 2, 1993

'The Treatment of 50 Cases of Premenstrual Breast Distension and Pain with *Jie Yu Huo Xue Tang* [Resolve Depression and Quicken the Blood Decoction]', Gu Si-yun, *Shan Dong Zhong Yi Za Zhi (Shandong Journal of Chinese Medicine)*, No. 6, 1992

'The Treatment of 24 Cases of Fibrocystic Breasts with *Ru Kuai Xiao Tang Jia Wei* [Breast Lump Dispersing Decoction with Added Flavours]', Hou Jian, *Shan Dong Zhong Yi Za Zhi (Shandong Journal of Chinese Medicine)*, No. 5, 1993

'The Treatment of 128 Cases of Fibrocystic Breasts', Mi Yang, *Hu Nan Zhong Yi Za Zhi (Hunan Journal of Chinese Medicine)*, No. 1, 1993

'Use of Basal Body Temperature in Pattern Discrimination for Patients with Infertility and Blocked Menstruation', Xia Gui-cheng, *Shang Hai Zhong Yi Yao Za Zhi (Shanghai Journal of Chinese Medicine and Medicinals)*, No. 10, 1992

Wan Shi Fu Ren Ke (Master Wan's Gynaecology), Wan Quan, a.k.a. Wan Mi-zhai, Hubei Science and Technology Press, 1984

Yi Zong Jin Jian (The Golden Mirror of Ancestral Medicine), Wu Qian *et al.*, People's Health and Hygiene Press, Beijing, 1985

Yu Xue Zheng Zhi (Static Blood Patterns and Treatments), Zhang Xue-wen, Shanxi Science and Technology Press, Xian, 1986

Zhen Jiu Da Cheng (A Great Compendium of Acupuncture and Moxibustion), Yang Ji-zhou, People's Health and Hygiene Press, Beijing, 1983

Zhen Jiu Xue (A Study of Acupuncture and Moxibustion), Qiu Mao-liang *et al.*, Shanghai Science and Technology Press, Shanghai, 1985

Zhen Jiu Yi Xue (An Easy Study of Acupuncture and Moxibustion), Li Shou-xian, People's Health and Hygiene Press, Beijing, 1990

Zhong Guo Min Jian Cao Yao Fang (Chinese Folk Herbal Medicinal Formulae), Liu Guang-rui and Liu Shao-lin, Sichuan Science and Technology Press, Chengdu, 1992

Zhong Guo Zhen Jiu Chu Fang Xue (A Study of Chinese Acupuncture and Moxibustion Prescriptions), Xiao Shao-qing, Ningxia People's Press, Yinchuan, 1986

Zhong Guo Zhong Yi Mi Fang Da Quan (A Great Compendium of Chinese National Chinese Medical Secret Formulae), Hu Zhao-ming (ed), Literary Propagation Publishing Company, Shanghai, 1992

Zhong Yi Fu Chan Ke Xue (A Study of Chinese Medical Gynaecology and Obstetrics), Heilonjiang College of TCM, People's Health and Hygiene Press, Beijing, 1991

Zhong Yi Fu Ke (Chinese Medical Gynaecology), Zhu Cheng-han, People's Heath and Hygiene Press, Beijing, 1989

Zhong Yi Fu Ke Lin Chuan Shou Ce (A Clinical Handbook of Chinese Medical Gynaecology), Shen Chong-li, Shanghai Science and Technology Press, Shanghai, 1990

Zhong Yi Fu Ke Shou Ce (A Handbook of Chinese Medical Gynaecology), Song Guang-ji and Yu Xiao-zhen, Zhejiang Science and Technology Press, Hangzhou, 1984; available in English, fourth, revised edition, trans. Zhang Ting-liang and Bob Flaws, Blue Poppy Press, Boulder, Colorado, 1995

Zhong Yi Fu Ke Xue (A Study of Chinese Medical Gynaecology), Chengdu College of Chinese Medicine, Shanghai Science and Technology Press, Shang-hai, 1983

Zhong Yi Fu Ke Xue (A Study of Chinese Medical Gynaecology), Liu Min-ru, Sichuan Science and Technology Press, Chengdu, 1992

Zhong Yi Fu Ke Xue (A Study of Chinese Medical Gynaecology), Luo Yuan-qi, Shanghai Science and Technology Press, Shanghai, 1987

Zhong Yi Fu Ke Zhi Liao Shou Ce (A Handbook of Chinese Medical Gynaecological Treatment), Wu Shi-xing and Qi Cheng-lin, Shan Xi Science and Technology Press, Xian, 1991

Zhong Yi Hu Li Xue (A Study of Chinese Medical Nursing), Lu Su-ying, People's Health and Hygiene Press, Beijing, 1983

Zhong Yi Lin Chuang Ge Ke (Various Clinical Specialities in Chinese Medicine), Zhang En-qin *et al.*, Shanghai College of TCM Press, Shanghai, 1990

Zhong Yi Ling Yan Fang (Efficacious Chinese Medical Formulae), Lin Bin-zhi, Science and Technology Propagation Press, Beijing, 1991

Zhong Yi Zhi Liao Fu Nu Bing (The Chinese Medical Treatment of Gynaecological Diseases), Zhang Jian-xiu, Hebei Science and Technology Press, 1988

Zhong Yi Zi Xue Cong Shu (The Chinese Medicine Self-study Series), Vol. 1, Gynaecology, Yang Yi-ya, Hebei Science and Technology Press, Shijiazhuang, 1987

ENGLISH LANGUAGE SOURCES

A Barefoot Doctor's Manual, revised and enlarged edition, Cloudburst Press, Mayne Isle, 1977

A Clinical Guide to Chinese Herbs and Formulae, Cheng Song-yu and Li Fei, Churchill and Livingstone, Edinburgh, 1993

A Compendium of TCM Patterns and Treatments, Bob Flaws and Daniel Finney, Blue Poppy Press, Boulder, Colorado, 1996

A Comprehensive Guide to Chinese Herbal Medicine, Chen Ze-lin and Chen Mei-fang, Oriental Healing Arts Institute, Long Beach, California, 1992

Arisal of the Clear: A Simple Guide to Healthy Eating According to Traditional Chinese Medicine, Bob Flaws, Blue Poppy Press, Boulder, Colorado, 1991

A Handbook of Differential Diagnosis with Key Signs and Symptoms, Therapeutic Principles and Guiding Prescriptions, Ou-yang Yi, trans. C.S. Cheung, Harmonious Sunshine Cultural Center, San Francisco, 1987

Chinese–English Terminology of Traditional Chinese Medicine, Shuai Xue-zhong *et al.*, Hunan Science and Technology Press, Changsha, 1983

Chinese–English Manual of Commonly Used Prescriptions in Traditional Chinese Medicine, Ou Ming (ed.), Joint Publishing Co. Ltd, Hong Kong, 1989

Chinese Herbal Medicine: Formulae and Strategies, Dan Bensky and Randall Barolet, Eastland Press, Seattle, 1990

Chinese Herbal Medicine: Materia Medica, Dan Bensky and Andrew Gamble, second, revised edition, Eastland Press, Seattle, 1993

Chinese Self-massage: The Easy Way to Health, Fan Ya-li, Blue Poppy Press, Boulder, Colorado, 1996

Chong and Ren Imbalance, Cyclic Management of Menstrual Disorders, Cheng Jing, trans. C.S. Cheung, Harmonious Sunshine Cultural Center, California, undated

Concise Traditional Chinese Gynaecology, Xia Gui-cheng *et al.,* Jiangsu Science and Technology Press, Nanjing, 1988

English–Chinese Chinese–English Dictionary of Chinese Medicine, Nigel Wiseman, Hunan Science and Technology Press, Changsha, 1995

Fundamentals of Chinese Acupuncture, Andrew Ellis, Nigel Wiseman and Ken Boss, Paradigm Publications, Brookline, Massachusetts, 1988

Fundamentals of Chinese Medicine, Nigel Wiseman and Andrew Ellis, Paradigm Publications, Brookline, Massachusetts, 1985

Glossary of Chinese Medical Terms and Acupuncture Points, Nigel Wiseman and Ken Boss, Paradigm Publications, Brookline, Massachusetts, 1990

Gynaecology and Obstetrics: A Longitudinal Approach, Thomas R. Moore *et al.* (eds.), Churchill Livingstone, New York, 1993

Handbook of Chinese Herbs and Formulae, Him-che Yeung, self-published, California, 1985

'Is Natural Progesterone the Missing Link in Osteoporosis Prevention and Treatment?', J. R. Lee, *Medical Hypotheses,* No. 35, 1991

'Menopausal Hormone Replacement Therapy with Continuous Daily Oral Micronized Estradiol and Progesterone', Joel T. Hargrove *et al., Gynaecology and Obstetrics,* Vol. 73, No. 4, April 1989

Oriental Materia Medica: A Concise Guide, Hong-yen Hsu, Oriental Healing Arts Institute, Long Beach, California, 1986

'Osteoporosis Reversal: The Role of Progesterone', John R. Lee, *International Clinical Nutrition Review,* Vol. 10, No. 3, July 1990

Practical Traditional Chinese Medicine and Pharmacology: Clinical Experiences, Shang Xian-min *et al.,* New World Press, Beijing, 1990

Practical Traditional Chinese Medicine and Pharmacology: Herbal Formulae, Geng Jun-ying *et al.,* New World Press, Beijing, 1991

'Progesterone and Its Relevance for Osteoporosis', Jerilynn C. Prior, *Osteoporosis,* Vol. 2, No. 2, March 1993

'Progesterone and the Prevention of Osteoporosis', Jerilynn C. Prior *et al.*, *The Canadian Journal of Obstetrics and Gynaecology and Women's Health Care*, Vol. 3, No. 4, 1991

'Progesterone as a Bone-trophic Hormone', J.C. Prior, *Endocrine Reviews*, Vol. 11, No. 2, 1990

'Spinal Bone Loss and Ovulatory Disturbances', Jerilynn C. Prior *et al.*, *The New England Journal of Medicine*, Volume 323, No. 18, November 1, 1990

Symptoms and Treatment for Menses and Leukorrhoea, Chen Yu-cang, trans. Hor Ming Lee, Hor Ming Press, Victoria, British Columbia, undated, a translation of *Jing Dai Zheng Zhi (Menstrual and Vaginal Discharge Patterns and Treatments)*

The English–Chinese Encyclopedia of Practical Traditional Chinese Medicine, Vol. 12: Gynaecology, Xuan Jia-sheng (ed.), Higher Education Press, Beijing, 1990

The Essential Book of Traditional Chinese Medicine, Vol. 2: Clinical Practice, Liu Yan-chi, trans. Fang Ting-yu and Chen Lai-di, Columbia University Press, New York, 1988

The Merck Manual of Diagnosis and Therapy, 15th edition, Robert Berkow (ed.), Merck Sharp and Dohme Research Laboratories, Rahway, New Jersey, 1987

The Nanjing Seminars Transcript, Qiu Mao-lian and Su Xu-ming, The Journal of Chinese Medicine, UK, 1985

'The Role of the Liver in Menstrual Disorders', (Rona) Wang Ru and Brian May, *The Pacific Journal of Oriental Medicine*, Australia, No. 77

The Treatise on the Spleen and Stomach, Li Dong-yuan, trans. Yang Shou-zhong, Blue Poppy Press, Boulder, Colorado 1993

'The Treatment of Fibrocystic Breast Disease with Chinese Herbs and Acupuncture', Deng Hui-ying and Liu Xin-ya, *The Journal of Chinese Medicine*, UK, No. 52, September 1996

The Yeast Connection, William G. Crook, Vintage Books, Random House, New York, 1986

The Yeast Syndrome, John Parks Towbridge and Morton Walker, Bantam Books, Toronto, 1988

Traditional Medicine in Contemporary China, Nathan Sivin, University of Michigan, Ann Arbor, 1987

Zang Fu: The Organ Systems of Traditional Chinese Medicine, second edition, Jeremy Ross, Churchill Livingstone, Edinburgh, 1985

INDEX

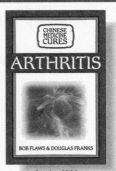

ARTHRITIS

BOB FLAWS & DOUGLAS FRANKS

October 1999 -
Chinese Medicine Cures Arthritis -
ISBN: 0-572-02540-8

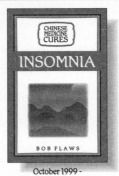

INSOMNIA

BOB FLAWS

October 1999 -
Chinese Medicine Cures Insomnia -
ISBN: 0-572-02568-8

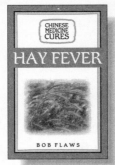

HAY FEVER

BOB FLAWS

February 2000 -
Chinese Medicine Cures Hayfever -
ISBN: 0-572-02576-9

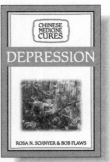

DEPRESSION

ROSA N. SCHNYER & BOB FLAWS

February 2000 -
Chinese Medicine Cures Depression -
ISBN: 0-572-02577-7

CHINESE
MEDICINE
CURES

BY WORLD-RENOWNED EXPERT
BOB FLAWS
Governor of the National Academy of
Acupuncture and Oriental Medicine
Fellow of The Register of
Chinese Herbal Medicine.
Edited by
Sylvia Schroer BSc MRCHM MBAcC
Council Member of the
Register of Chinese Medicine

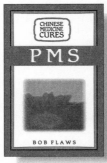

PMS

BOB FLAWS

Summer 2000 -
Chinese Medicine Cures PMS - ISBN:
0-572-02539-4

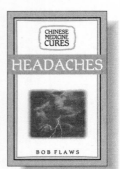

HEADACHES

BOB FLAWS

Summer 2000 -
Chinese Medicine Cures Headaches -
ISBN: 0-572-02590-4

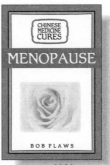

MENOPAUSE

BOB FLAWS

Autumn 2000 -
Chinese Medicine Cures Menopause -
ISBN: 0-572-02591-2

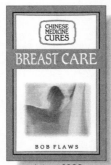

BREAST CARE

BOB FLAWS

Autumn 2000 -
Chinese Medicine Cures Breast Care-
ISBN: 0-572-02592-0